Dravet Syndrome

Topics in Epilepsy series, vol. 3

ISBN: 978-2-7420-0737-0

Published by

Éditions John Libbey Eurotext

127, avenue de la République, 92120 Montrouge, France

Tel.: +33 (0)1 46 73 06 60

Website: www.jle.com

John Libbey Eurotext

42-46 High Street,

Esther, Surrey,

KT10 9KY

United Kingdom

Dravet Syndrome

Authors
Charlotte Dravet, Renzo Guerrini

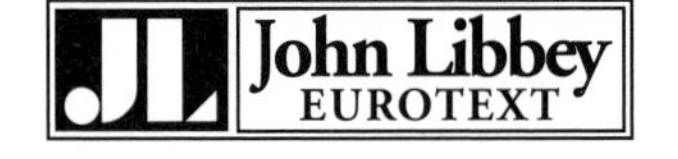

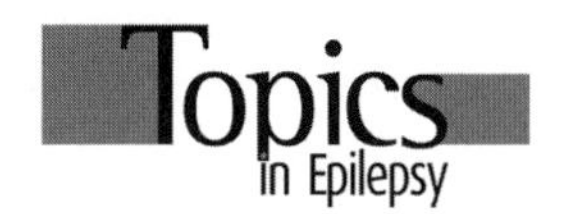

Foreword

Dravet Syndrome is one of the best examples of a successful cooperation between clinicians, neurophysiologists and geneticists, developed and progressively intensified during the last thirty years. It also represents a very convincing example of how the syndromic approach to the epilepsies, promoted by the Marseille school under the cultural and scientific leadership of J. Roger and C.A. Tassinari, is a winning approach.

In fact Dravet Syndrome, as currently known, originates from the initial identification of a well defined and easily recognizable electroclinical entity characterized by a peculiar fever sensitivity, called Severe Myoclonic Epilepsy of Infancy (SMEI) because of its early onset, strong myoclonic component and poor prognosis.

SMEI has been identified as a result of a "splitting" operation on a population of subjects with a suspicious diagnosis of Lennox-Gastaut syndrome (mainly at the Centre St Paul of Marseille) and on a population with myoclonic epilepsy or febrile seizures starting in the first 3 years of life (mainly at the Child Neuropsychiatry Unit in Verona).

This "splitting" approach was based on the analysis of repeated clinical and EEG-polygraphic or video-EEG-polygraphic assessments that, collected throughout evolution, allowed to identify the electroclinical phenotype of SMEI.

In the following years, thanks to the continuous and passionate work of divulgation in the world done by C. Dravet, the clinical studies lead to the documentation of a wider electro-clinical phenotype spectrum with a common genetic denominator, and the term SMEI was replaced by Dravet Syndrome.

The merit of this book is to be a timely and masterly description of the multifaceted electro-clinical, genetics and evolutive aspects of the Dravet Syndrome.

For the clinician the book is very interesting and easy to read because of the quality of the text and of its structure. Thank to the collaborative work of C. Dravet and R. Guerrrini, description and documentation of the electroclinical features are very good and will certainly help a correct diagnosis, the best available treatment options are fully illustrated and current knowledge of the syndrome's genetics is thoroughly updated.

The only big limit of the book, obviously not imputable to the Authors, is given by the vast amount of questions that, in spite of current knowledge, remain unanswered. What are the real nosological limits of the syndrome? Are there real genotype-phenotype correlations? Which elements determine the evolution of epilepsy and, in particular, of developmental impairment? Which parameters hold a predictive value for prognosis? And, consequently, what is the best treatment strategy?

The present contribution, documenting the great variability of evolution and of the response to therapy, consequent to the increasing widening of the syndrome spectrum, points out the limits of current knowledge. Therefore the present contribution, beyond giving an excellent update of the present knowledge on Dravet Syndrome, evidences with lucidity and honesty what is still unknown and sends an invitation to multiply the efforts in this direction.

Probably, considering that even genetic diagnosis is of little use to predict the severity of the disorder, following the "lumping" operation which lead to the Dravet Syndrome, now it is time again for a "splitting" approach. Obviously not in order to break up Dravet Syndrome but in order to recognize those electroclinical spectrum features having a sound prognostic meaning.

New electroclinical longitudinal studies considering, jointly from the onset, clinical, video-EEG-polygraphic and developmental aspects within the different treatment responses, might allow recognising different subsyndrome aggregations of manifestations, having prognostic value, perhaps related to genetic variability.

This book other than documenting the continuous, passionate and fruitful effort of Charlotte Dravet in this field, will be a very useful instrument for all the people involved in the difficult task of diagnosis, treatment and management of children with epilepsy.

Bernardo Dalla Bernardina

Direttore di dipartimento Neuropsichiatria Infantile, Azienda Ospedaliera di Verona, Italy.

Content

« Les mères en savent plus sur les convulsions que les médecins, je crois.
[...] Je te le répète, une seule chose est certaine :
voir son enfant en convulsion, voilà l'enfer pour une mère. »
Honoré de Balzac. *La Comédie humaine* (1841).

« Mothers, it is my belief, know more than doctors do about convulsions.
[...] One thing alone, as I said before, is certain,
that it is hell for a mother to see her child in convulsions. »
The Human Comedy, by Honoré de Balzac (1841).

Introduction

"Severe myoclonic epilepsy in infancy" is a type of epilepsy first described in 1978, in patients examined at Marseille by Charlotte Dravet. At that time, many children with severe epilepsy and cognitive impairment were diagnosed with Lennox-Gastaut syndrome and were admitted to the Centre Saint-Paul. An accurate observation of seizures and electroencephalograms, as well as detailed history taking, led to the recognition that, in some of these children, epilepsy could not be diagnosed as Lennox-Gastaut syndrome and was characterised by common features, particularly onset in the first year of life, fever sensitivity and myoclonic seizures. Bernardo Dalla Bernardina, who worked simultaneously in Verona, Italy, and at the centre Saint-Paul, also observed the same electroclinical features in his Italian patients. Subsequently, C. Dravet, M. Bureau, B. Dalla Bernardina and J. Roger presented these patients at the XIIIth International Epilepsy Congress, in Kyoto, in 1982.

Later, more cases were described from other countries and it became clear that these patients had a newly recognised epilepsy syndrome, which also implied some variability. A lack of myoclonic seizures in a subset of patients and the persistence of epilepsy into adulthood led to the name "Dravet syndrome" instead of "severe myoclonic epilepsy in infancy".

Given the absence of a recognisable aetiology, the relatively high incidence of epilepsy and febrile seizures in the family members, we suspected a genetic origin to the syndrome. It was the seizure-precipitating role of fever that prompted the Belgium team of Antwerp to look for a mutation in the same gene which may be mutated in patients with GEFS+, particularly since cases of Dravet syndrome had been reported in families with GEFS+. A mutation in *SCN1A* was identified in all the seven patients tested. Since this time, the syndrome has been extensively studied by geneticists and has become a model for epilepsies caused by channelopathies. R. Guerrini and co-workers, in Florence, Italy, contributed to the knowledge of the genetic basis and response to antiepileptic drugs of Dravet syndrome.

An animal model, a mutant mouse, was created through experimental research from independent laboratories and is essential for the progression of our understanding of the mechanisms at stake in this epilepsy and identification of new therapeutic targets.

Advances in treatment are encouraging as new molecules have emerged that allow a better control of seizures and a striking decrease in the episodes of status epilepticus. Early mortality, often due to sudden unexpected death in epilepsy (SUDEP) has been recognized as a significant concern but has not been accurately studied. Studies on cognitive development have shown there is variability in the degree of impairment and outcome is not always as severe as described in first reports.

As Dravet syndrome is both rare and severe, families have felt isolated, needed to communicate with one another using internet forums, and thus involved themselves in national and international associations. Besides providing self help, these associations have contributed to a better knowledge of the syndrome for the neurological and paediatric communities and has stimulated scientific research.

In 2009, C. Dravet, M. Bureau, B. Dalla Bernardina and R. Guerrini *(Figure 1)* decided the time had come to present the state of current knowledge about this epilepsy type and organised an international workshop in Verona, Italy. The main contributions of this meeting were summarised in a supplement of *Epilepsia*.

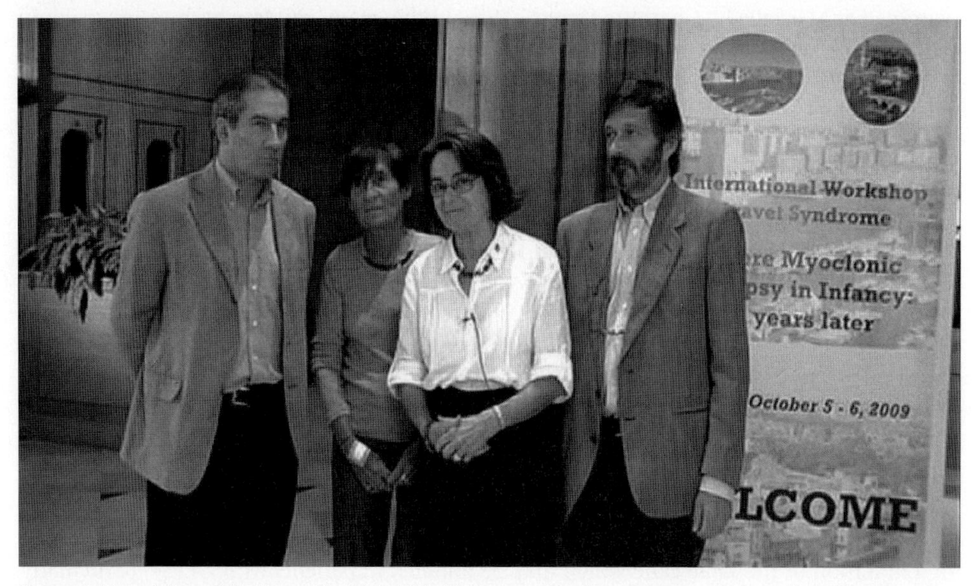

Figure 1. *From left to right: Renzo Guerrini, Michelle Bureau, Charlotte Dravet and Bernardo Dalla Bernardina.*

This book aims to provide more information on the syndrome to those neurologists, child neurologists, and paediatricians confronted with infants, children and adults who either have or are suspected to have Dravet syndrome. We are aware that significant gaps in our understanding of the syndrome remain, however, we hope this contribution may assist in the understanding of the disease and optimisation of treatments.

We express our warm thanks to our patients and their families for their confidence and collaboration, which is invaluable for the understanding of the disease. We admire how they take care of their children and strive to offer them the best possible quality of life. We thank all our co-workers in France and Italy, including those who participated in the multi-centre studies. We especially thank Bernardo Dalla Bernardina and Michelle Bureau who strongly contributed to the delineation of the syndrome and who are still deeply involved in the study of the syndrome. We also acknowledge Doctor Joseph Roger who was our mentor, as medical director of the Centre Saint-Paul, and maintained that good clinical practice goes hand in hand with a scientific approach. We are lastly grateful to the team of the Biocodex laboratory who opened the door for a better treatment of this epilepsy with the discovery of a new molecule with antiepileptic properties (stiripentol), which has changed the life of most affected families.

Charlotte Dravet,
Centre Saint-Paul, Hôpital Henri-Gastaut, Marseille, France.
Childhood Neuropsychiatry Unit, Policlinico A. Gemelli, Catholic University, Roma, Italy.

Renzo Guerrini,
Paediatric Neurology Unit and Laboratories, Children's Hospital A. Meyer, University of Florence, Firenze, Italy.

1. Historical, Definition, Epidemiology

Historical

Dravet syndrome (DS) is a rare form of epilepsy, accompanied by impaired psychomotor and neurological development, occurring in the first year of life in apparently normal infants. It was initially described in 1978, in a French medical journal (Dravet, 1978), under the name of "severe myoclonic epilepsy of infancy" (SMEI), in order to distinguish it from Lennox-Gastaut syndrome (LGS).

In the following years, at the Centre Saint-Paul in Marseille, C. Dravet collected 42 cases which were presented at the XIIIth Epilepsy International Symposium at Kyoto in 1982 (Dravet *et al.*, 1982). From this time, several authors reported similar cases in Europe and Japan (Dalla Bernardina *et al.*, 1982; Ogino *et al.*, 1985) and it became progressively obvious that these cases represented a subset of patients affected by the same epileptic syndrome. Thereafter, many children were reported to have symptoms similar to SMEI but without myoclonus (Sugama *et al.*, 1987; Ogino *et al.*, 1989; Kanazawa, 1992; Yakoub *et al.*, 1992; Dravet *et al.*, 1992a, 2005a, b). These patients may have different EEG features but they share the same course and outcome as those with myoclonus, and can be included in the same syndrome as *borderline forms* (SMEB). This observation seems to be supported by recent genetic studies which revealed a *SCN1A* gene mutation in patients with and without myoclonus (Fukuma *et al.*, 2004). Moreover, epilepsy was not limited to infancy and childhood and was reported to persist into adulthood. For these reasons, it was proposed that the name be changed to "severe polymorphic epilepsy of infants" (Aicardi, 1994) and subsequently to the eponym "Dravet syndrome".

In 1989, the revised classification of the International League Against Epilepsy placed SMEI under the heading of "epilepsies and syndromes undetermined as to whether they are focal or generalised," since the syndrome shows both generalised and localised seizure types and EEG paroxysms (Commission on Classification and Terminology of the International League Against Epilepsy, 1989).

In the scheme proposed by the ILAE (Engel, 2001), DS is considered as an "epileptic encephalopathy", defined as *"a condition in which the epileptiform abnormalities themselves are believed to contribute to the progressive disturbance in cerebral function"*. In 2010 (Berg *et al.*, 2010), this definition was slightly altered: *"the epileptic activity itself may contribute to severe cognitive and behavioural impairment above and beyond what might be expected from the underlying patho-*

logy alone (e.g. cortical malformation) and that these can worsen over time". The latter better corresponds to DS in which the cognitive decline observed in the first stages of the disease is probably due not only to epilepsy but also to genetic and environmental factors.

Definition

According to the ILAE classification (1989), typical DS is characterised by *"febrile and afebrile generalised and unilateral, clonic or tonic-clonic, seizures, that occur in the first year of life in an otherwise normal infant and are later associated with myoclonus, atypical absences, and partial seizures. All seizure types are resistant to antiepileptic drugs (AEDs). Developmental delay becomes apparent within the second year of life and is followed by definite cognitive impairment and personality disorders".*

Other features can be added. A family history of epilepsy or febrile seizures (FS) is frequently reported. A small elevation of temperature is sufficient to trigger convulsive seizures, usually in an infectious context. Clonic seizures have a tendency to become prolonged and evolve into status epilepticus. Unilateral seizures may involve both sides of the body, alternatively. Atypical absences can be prolonged and translate into obtundation status. Developmental delay is accompanied by behavioural disorders, such as hyperactivity, lack of attention, oppositive features and, less often, a tendency to withdraw. Neurological signs such as ataxia, interictal myoclonus of the extremities, and pyramidal signs can also occur in the second year. Interictal EEGs traces do not present with a typical pattern and are normal at the onset in most patients. Later on, they show generalised and multifocal abnormalities. Photosensitivity is frequent (49.2% in the Dravet series) and can be observed in the first year of life (Dravet *et al.*, 1992a). Neuroimaging and metabolic screening do not detect any anomaly.

A number of patients do not present with this full picture and are considered to have a borderline form of the syndrome (SMEB). They share the main characteristics for all of the features, except seizure type. Generalised and unilateral clonic and tonic-clonic seizures are always present, but myoclonic seizures and atypical absences are not observed, and focal seizures are inconstantly observed (Sugama *et al.*, 1987; Ogino *et al.*, 1989; Yakoub *et al.*, 1992). We have also described these incomplete forms (Dravet *et al.*, 1992a). Conversely, we did not observe the features of patients reported in Japan, with only generalised tonic-clonic seizures and a peculiar EEG pattern, described as *"childhood epilepsy with intractable grand mal seizures"* (Fujiwara *et al.*, 1992) or *"high voltage slow wave- grand mal syndrome"* (Kanazawa, 1992). Some of these patients also presented with hemiclonic and focal seizures and they shared the same course and outcome as other patients. In Germany, a larger group with *"severe idiopathic generalised epilepsy of infancy with generalised tonic-clonic seizures"* was reported (Doose *et al.*, 1998). This group was more heterogeneous and comprised patients who fulfilled the criteria for SMEI and others with only grand mal seizures, the onset age extending to 5 years.

The prognosis is unfavourable in almost all cases; seizures become drug-resistant and persist; all patients have motor and cognitive impairment, and early mortality rate is high (16-18%; Dravet *et al.*, 2005a, b).

Since 2001, it is known that in most cases the syndrome results from a *de novo* mutation of the *SCN1A* gene, which encodes the voltage-gated sodium channel Nav1.1 (Claes *et al.*, 2001). Most patients with a borderline form also carry mutations in the *SCN1A* gene (Ohmori *et al.*, 2003; Fujiwara *et al.*, 2003; Oguni *et al.*, 2005). It has been shown that 70% of the patients with SMEI or SMEB carry a *SCN1A* mutation, which is rarely inherited (Marini *et al.*, 2007). Many studies failed to find a significant correlation between genotype and phenotype (Ohmori *et al.*, 2003; Wallace *et al.*, 2003; Fukuma *et al.*, 2004; Oguni *et al.*, 2005), except an earlier age at onset in patients carrying a truncation, splice mutation or a genomic deletion compared to those with a missense mutation or without *SCN1A* mutation (Marini *et al.*, 2007).

As we consider DS and SMEI as two denominations of the same entity, we will use the synonymous terms. We will use the definition borderline forms (which are specified as SMEB or borderline DS) only when relevant differences from DS are apparent.

Epidemiology

DS is a rare disorder but its actual frequency is not well known. An incidence of probably less than 1 per 40,000 was reported in 1990 in the USA (Hurst, 1990). Slightly different figures (1/20,000 or 30,000) were reported in France by Yakoub *et al.* (1992). In these studies, males were more often affected than females in a ratio of 2:1. However, this ratio may not correspond to true values, since in the last study of a large cohort of 802 individuals realised by the International Dravet syndrome Epilepsy Action League (the IDEA League), the ratio was 1:1 (Skluzacek *et al.*, 2011).

The percentage of patients with SMEI, relative to patients with seizure onset in the first year of life, has been reported in two previous studies: Caraballo *et al.* (1997) identified 3% of patients with SMEI in a series of 471 patients between 1992 and 1997, and Yakoub *et al.* (1992) identified 5% among 329 patients between 1980 and 1985. In two other studies, 7% and 6.1% patients with SMEI were determined for patients with seizure onset before the age of three (Dalla Bernardina *et al.*, 1983; Dravet *et al.*, 1992a, respectively). Dravet *et al.* (2002) identified 445 published cases. Recently, in a Spanish population of 365 patients with epilepsy, aged from one month to less than 15 years, five patients were reported with DS (1.4%) (Durà-Travé *et al.*, 2007). The prevalence in the USA for the year 2008 was estimated at between 2,000 and 8,000 cases, in any instance lower than 10,000, based on expert opinion data that was submitted to the FDA to conclude that DS is rare in the US (Benjamin P. Lewis, Personal communication, Lewis Regulatory Consulting, LLC).

Thus, even if recognition of the syndrome has increased in the last decade, DS remains a rare disease. It is classified as ORPHA 33069 in the Orphanet classification.

2. Clinical and EEG Description

In collaboration with Michelle Bureau

Centre Saint-Paul, Hôpital Henri-Gastaut, Marseille, France

Spanish authors (Lambarri San Martin *et al.*, 1997) considered that the course of SMEI can be divided into three stages: a "febrile phase" in the first year, a "catastrophic phase" of variable duration, and a "sequel phase". We agree with this description but are reluctant to use the term "catastrophic" which is too impressive for families and thus prefer the term "worsening phase". Likewise, we prefer the term "stabilisation" to "sequel" because epilepsy remains active in the third phase. However, in this chapter, we will not use this distinction in phases since the age limits between the second and third phase are unclear; instead, the onset and steady state are considered and there is a separate chapter for long-term outcome.

Onset

Age at onset

Severe myoclonic epilepsy begins during the first year of life. All authors report a mean onset age of between five and eight months *(Table I)*. Only two authors (Hurst, 1987; Kearney *et al.*, 2006) reported three patients who presented a first seizure after one year (at 13, 16 and 18 months, respectively).

Family history

A large proportion of cases have a family history of epilepsy or FS, but this is difficult to estimate with any accuracy because of the high variability between studies; from around 25% in initial series to 50% or higher in the most recent series (71% in the study of Ohki *et al.* [1997] and 46% in the study of Ragona *et al.* [2010]). In these studies, a relationship with genetic alterations was not investigated. In a recent study on a homogeneous group of patients bearing *SCN1A* mutations (Mancardi *et al.*, 2006), the authors found 27% of patients with a family history of seizures. Based on a series of 96 patients with FS in the first year of life, Hattori *et al.* (2008) showed that a family history was present for 28% of patients with DS and 50% for non-DS patients. However, in another study (Marini *et al.*, 2007) the rate of family history of seizures was 54.5% in the whole group, 51.2% in patients with SCN1A mutations, and 62.5% in those without a mutation.

Table I. *Age at seizure onset in the literature.*

Author	Age	
	Mean	Range
Akiyama *et al.*, 2010	5 m	2-7 m
Korff *et al.*, 2007	5 m 4 d	3-10 m
Dravet *et al.*, 1992	5 m 6 d	2-9 m
Dulac & Arthuis, 1982	5 m 7 d	3-8 m
Ragona *et al.*, 2010	5 m 7 d	3-11 m
Dalla Bernardina *et al.*, 1982	6 m	
Caraballo & Fejerman, 2006	6 m	3-12 m
Aicardi & Levi Gomes, 1989	6 m 27 d	
Hurst, 1987	8 m 4 d	4-18 m

Few authors have separated FS from epilepsy in the family histories. In the study of Nieto-Barrera *et al.* (2000a), 21% of families had FS and 32% had epilepsy, of which two families had both. Dravet *et al.* (2005a, b) reported 16.6% with FS and 20% with epilepsy, of which three families had both. Parents' consanguinity was noted in three cases. In the Tokyo study (Oguni *et al.*, 2001), there were 27.3% with FS and 14.2% with epilepsy. When indicated, the epilepsy type in families is idiopathic generalised epilepsy (Dalla Bernardina *et al.*, 1982; Benloumis *et al.*, 2001; Ragona *et al.*, 2010).

At least 13 families with two affected siblings have been reported (Ogino *et al.*, 1989; Dravet *et al.*, 1992a; Veggiotti *et al.*, 2001; Gennaro *et al.*, 2003, 2006; Kimura *et al.*, 2005; Morimoto *et al.*, 2006; Depienne *et al.*, 2006; Marini *et al.*, 2007). In two families, one sibling had a typical form and the other a borderline form. Fujiwara *et al.* (2003) reported two families with two affected siblings; in the first family, the sister had SMEI and her brother had febrile seizures; in the second family, the sister had SMEI and her brother had partial epilepsy. No further details were provided.

Seven pairs of affected twins have been reported: five pairs were monozygotic twins (Fujiwara *et al.*, 1990, 1992; Musumecci *et al.*, 1992; Ohki *et al.*, 1997; Miyama *et al.*, 2008), one pair were dizygotic (Ohtsuka *et al.*, 1991), and the remaining unknown (Jansen *et al.*, 2006).

Personal antecedents and associated pathology

Infants do not usually have a personal pathological history preceding seizure onset. However, for 22% of patients in our first series (Dravet *et al.*, 1992a), we noted more or less relevant antecedents during pregnancy and delivery. Surprisingly, this rate was higher in two series; at 66% for Giovanardi-Rossi *et al.* (1991) and 40% for Ragona *et al.* (2010).

• In three patients, DS was associated with a genetic disease: Rud syndrome (Musumeci *et al.*, 1992), epidermal naevus syndrome and type I neurofibromatosis (Dravet *et al.*, 2005a, b). No genetic analysis was performed in these patients.

• Congenital cardiac defect are not reported in the literature but we have identified one unpublished patient carrying a tricuspid valve atresia and are aware of other cases reported by families.

• We are also aware of two unrelated children suffering from a growth hormone deficit.

• A girl with SMEI was a member of a family with GEFS+ (published in Depienne *et al.*, 2010) of which several members, including the proband, had haemophilia due to a deficit in factor VIII.

Physical and psychomotor development is apparently normal.

Clinical semiology at onset

The first seizure is typically clonic, generalised or unilateral, triggered by fever but often longer than a simple febrile seizure. Several Japanese authors (Sugama *et al.*, 1987; Fujiwara *et al.*, 1990) have underlined the triggering effect of Japanese-style hot water immersion, which produces body temperature elevation (see below).

However, variations in the mode of onset have been observed by all authors. Convulsive seizures can occur without fever in 28% (Ohki *et al.*, 1997) to 35% (Dravet *et al.*, 2005a, b) and 61% (Ragona *et al.*, 2010) of the children. In our series, these afebrile seizures usually occurred in the context of a vaccination or infectious episode, or after a bath. Later on, afebrile seizures were associated with febrile seizures in 80% of patients. Nieto-Barrera *et al.* (2000a) emphasized the coincidence between the first seizure and DTP vaccination.

These seizures, with or without fever, tend to be long and last for more than 20 minutes for 25% (Dravet *et al.*, 2005a, b) to 49% (Ragona *et al.*, 2010) of the patients, and to evolve into status epilepticus. The first seizures can be focal. In some patients, isolated episodes of focal myoclonic jerking are noted by the parents, in the absence of fever, either some weeks or some days before the appearance of the first convulsive seizure. These episodes remain isolated or occur in the hours preceding the first convulsive seizure, repetitively, together with hyperthermia. Complex partial seizures can also be observed (the literature includes two cases by Dravet *et al.* [2005a, b], at least five cases by Oguni *et al.* [2001], and one case by Ohki *et al.* [1997]). Recently, Hino-Fukuyo *et al.* (2009) reported focal seizures with ictal vomiting as the initial seizures in two twins. Actually, the first seizure was a convulsive status epilepticus, without vomiting, however, in their subsequent episodes, vomiting was always the initial symptom, followed by febrile and non-febrile convulsions lasting from five to 30 minutes.

Ragona *et al.* (2010) observed variation in initial seizures according to the age at onset. These seizures had a tendency to be longer when they occurred before the age of six months, with status epilepticus in 11 of 27 patients, whereas they were shorter when they occurred after six months, with status epilepticus in only three of 10 patients. However, this difference was not statistically significant.

EEG semiology at onset

At onset, background activity while awake is usually normal for age. In some cases, a rhythmic theta activity of 4-5 Hz is noted over the rolandic and vertex areas (Dalla Bernardina *et al.*, 1982; Giovanardi-Rossi *et al.*, 1991). The sleep EEG shows normal organisation with physiological patterns for age. A diffuse or unilateral slowing of the background activity may be observed if the EEG is realised shortly after a prolonged seizure.

In around 20 to 25% of cases, generalised spike-waves (SWs) are elicited by intermittent photic stimulation, a most unusual finding at that age (Dalla Bernardina *et al.*, 1982; Dravet *et al.*, 1992a).

The first seizure is often considered as a FS, few investigations are performed and no treatment is given. However, shortly thereafter, other febrile seizures occur (two weeks to two months, mean: six weeks [Dulac & Arthuis, 1982]) and afebrile seizures also appear (two months to 14 months, mean: five months [Ohki *et al.*, 1997]). Between one and four years old, other seizure types appear, simultaneously with a slowing of psychomotor development and the picture becomes characteristic of a steady state.

Steady State

Steady state: Seizures

Patients with SMEI have multiple seizure types during the course of the disease:
- convulsive seizures consisting of generalised tonic-clonic (GTCS), or generalised clonic seizures (GCS), or alternating unilateral clonic seizures,
- myoclonic seizures,
- atypical absences and obtundation status,
- focal seizures: simple focal motor seizures and complex partial seizures, with or without secondary generalisation,
- rarely, tonic seizures.

The following descriptions are mainly based on the data of a study conducted in Marseille on 60 patients whose seizures were carefully analysed by video-polygraphic EEG recordings. These data are compared with those in the literature.

Convulsive seizures

These are present throughout life in all patients. We use this term to group all seizures, apparently generalised or unilateral, which are usually classified as tonic-clonic or clonic.

However, the Marseille study demonstrated, in many cases, peculiar clinical and EEG features which precluded them from being classified as true generalised seizures. Most seizures were recorded during sleep, either nocturnal or diurnal, at various stages of the course, usually after the age of three. We have tried to group the seizures by distinguishing several different forms: apparently true generalised clonic or tonic-clonic seizures (nine patients), unilateral seizures (nine patients), "falsely generalised" seizures (10 patients), and "unstable" seizures (11 patients). In fact, this distinction of subtypes is somewhat artificial and all these seizures, except generalised seizures, seem to belong to the same category of seizures with focal onset and rapid spread to the adjacent areas or opposite hemisphere. Furthermore, they can occur in association in the same patient.

Generalised convulsions (recorded in nine cases). These resemble the GTCS of the idiopathic generalised epilepsies. However, they are usually shorter, with a very brief tonic phase, few autonomic symptoms, and a transient postictal flattening which is rapidly replaced by diffuse delta waves. These characteristics are those observed in the GTCS in childhood *(Figure 2)*. In some seizures, the initial tonic phase is almost immediately mixed with the clonic jerks, giving a vibratory aspect which is well documented in the three cases published by Ogihara *et al.* (1994).

We did not record seizures described as clonic-tonic-clonic convulsions by Fujiwara *et al.* (1992) and reported in two patients by Ohki *et al.* (1997), in which a short clonic phase precedes the tonic phase. Thus, we do not believe this type of seizure is typical of DS.

Unilateral seizures. True hemiclonic seizures, corresponding to the description by Gastaut *et al.* (1974), have been recorded only in two young children (16 months and three years, respectively) in our series of 60 patients. They became less common with age, as also mentioned by Ohki *et al.* (1997). Ragona *et al.* (2010) reported unilateral seizures in 14 of 37 patients in the first year of life. However, there were other unilateral seizures (in seven patients) with different characteristics, including: shorter duration, association with contralateral tonus changes, and ictal EEG abnormalities more limited to one hemisphere.

In all cases, there are postictal asymmetric EEG signs and, often, a postictal transitory hemiparesis. These seizures can be either on one side or on the contralateral side in the same patient, this alternating pattern being a clue for the diagnosis of SMEI. *(Figure 3 a, b)*. The localised origin of unilateral seizures often goes unnoticed. The unilateral seizures are rarely described by other authors who, probably, consider it to be focal. Caraballo & Fejerman (2006) reported one child who presented with a severe focal status epilepticus and developed hemiparesis with contralateral cerebral hemiatrophy, confirmed by CT and MRI scans. This type of outcome is similar to that which occurs after a hemiclonic seizure (Gastaut *et al.*, 1974). We observed

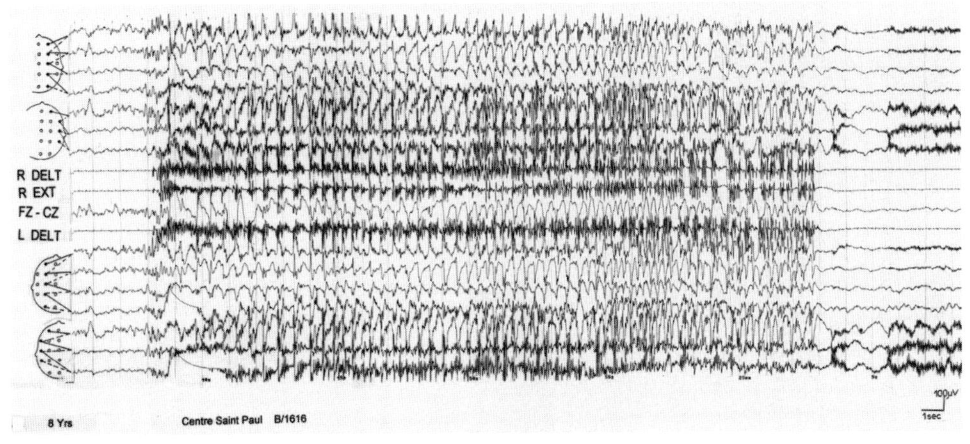

Figure 2. *Generalised tonic-clonic seizure in a eight-year-old boy.*
At onset: *brief burst of fast activity (less than 1 s) progressively intermixed with slow waves. The end of the seizure is marked by a brief flattening followed by low voltage theta activity. The EMG recorded over the 2 deltoids shows a tonic contraction followed by sustended myoclonias which become irregular and very fast, with a vibratory aspect.*
R DELT = right deltoid muscle; R EXT = right wrist extensor muscle; L DELT = left deltoid muscle.

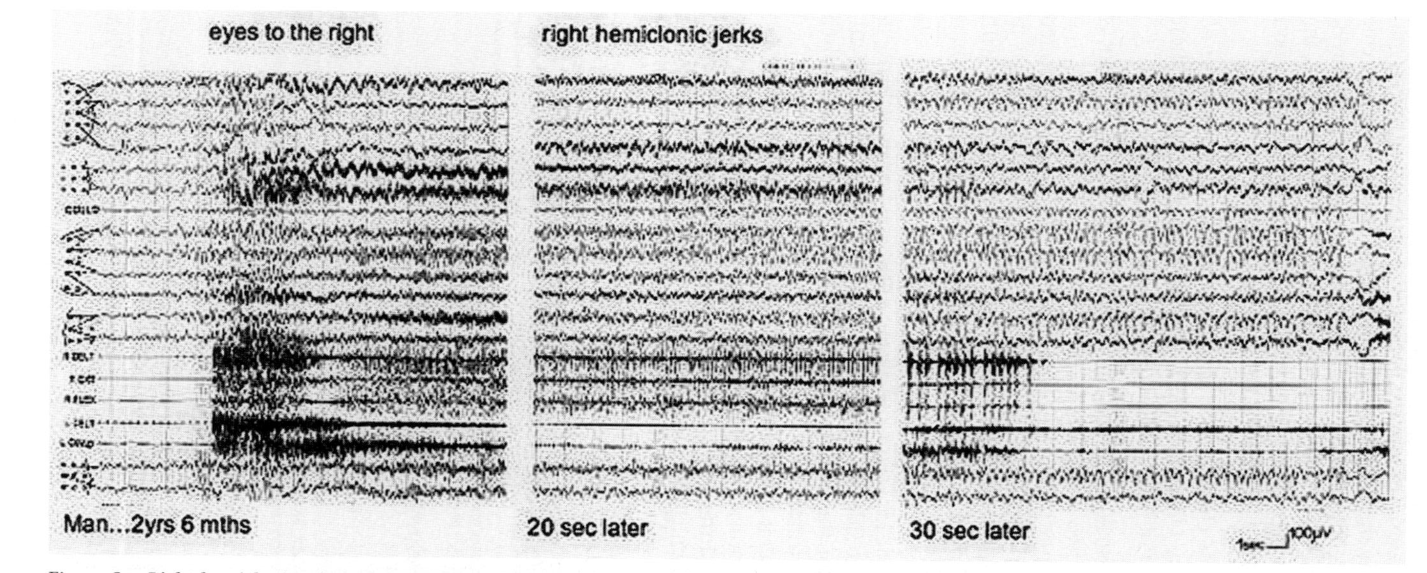

Figure 3a. *Right hemiclonic seizure in a two-and-a-half-year-old boy during epileptic status.*

Left: *On the left hemisphere, slow waves and spikes followed by high-voltage fast activity. On the right hemisphere theta activity with muscular artefacts over the temporal area due to the head and mouth deviation to the right. On the polygraphy, at onset diffuse tonic contraction, then vibratory phase on the right muscles.*

Middle: *20 s later, rhythmic diffuse discharge of spikes and waves on the left hemisphere, predominantly on the anterior area, spreading discretely to the right anterior region, accompanied by rhythmic clonic jerks on the right side of the body.*

Right: *30 s later: the discharge on the left hemisphere slows down, still spreading on the right and ceases abruptly, followed by a left flattening and a right hemiparesis. Note that the right myoclonic jerks cease before the end of the EEG discharge.*

R DELT = right deltoid muscle; R EXT = right wrist extensor muscle; R FLEX = right wrist flexor muscle; L DELT = left deltoid muscle; L QUAD = left quadriceps muscle; oculo = oculogramme.

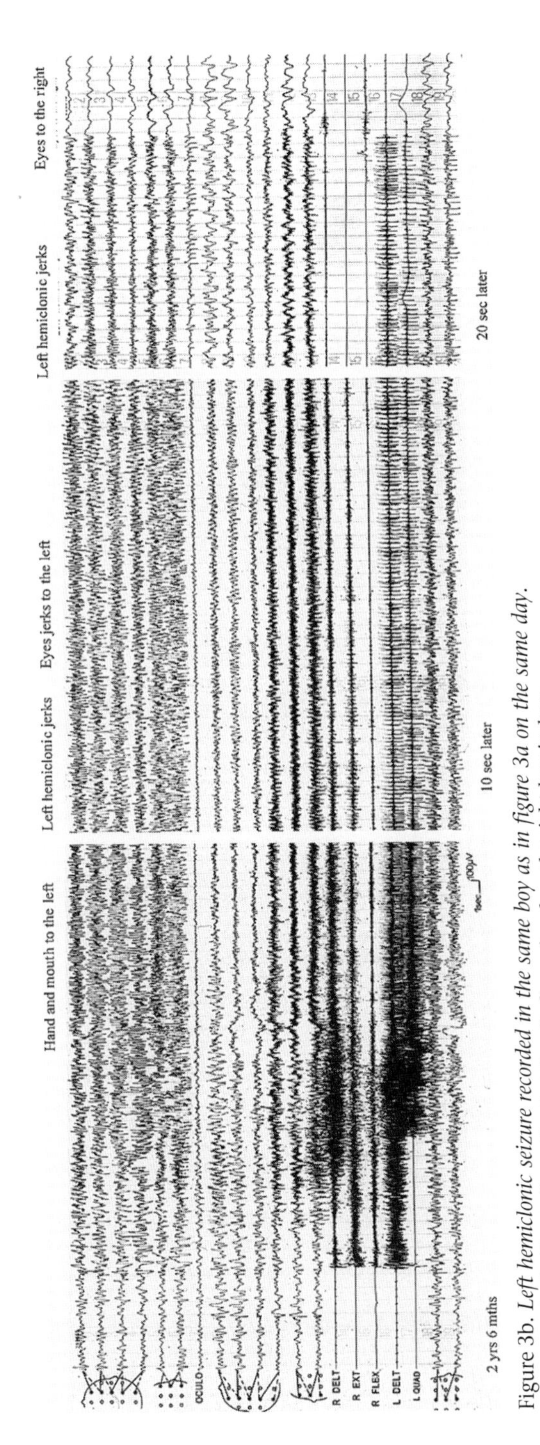

Figure 3b. *Left hemiclonic seizure recorded in the same boy as in figure 3a on the same day. The aspect is similar to figure 2a, but the discharge involves the right hemisphere.*
R DELT = right deltoid muscle; R EXT = right wrist extensor muscle; R FLEX = right wrist flexor muscle; L DELT = left deltoid muscle; L QUAD = left quadriceps muscle; oculo = oculogramme.

one three-year-old girl who had a right hemiclonic seizure at home. When she arrived at the emergency room the seizure was over and the girl was conscious but slightly obnubilated, with perioral myoclonia and right hemiparesis. At this time, the EEG showed continuous left hemispheric slow waves and SWs, which lasted until lorazepam was *i.v.* injected *(Figure 4).*

"Falsely generalised seizures" (recorded in 10 cases). These are characterised by a complex semiology with some degree of discrepancy between clinical and EEG phenomena.

Parents report these seizures as GTCS. But, accurate observation by video-polygraphic EEG recording demonstrates that they are not primarily generalised and are different from one patient to another. They usually consist of a bilateral, asymmetric, tonic contraction, leading to

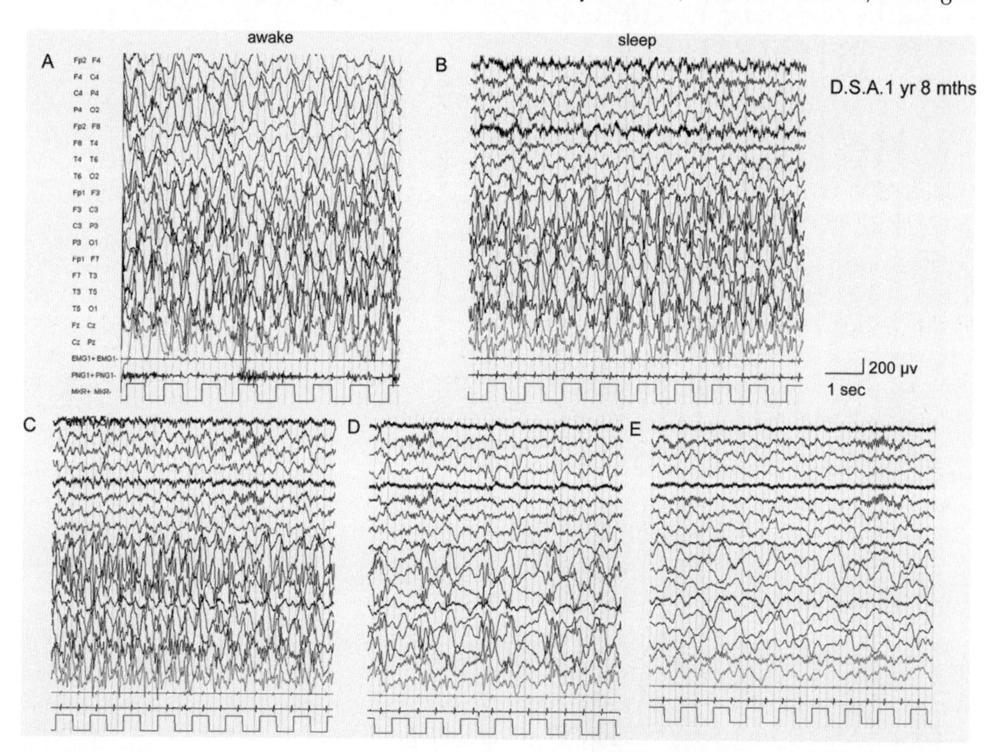

Figure 4. *EEG recording four hours after the clinical end of a right hemiclonic seizure in a one-year, eight-month-old girl.*
This 1 year 8 month-old girl had a right hemiclonic seizure which lasted more than 30 m and was interrupted by rectal diazepam, and followed by a right hemiparesis.
A and B: *awake and sleep EEG recording 4 hours after the end of the hemiclonic seizure. In A, the girl being drowsy, without clinical seizure, spikes, poly-spikes and slow waves on the left hemisphere and delta waves on the right. In B, during sleep, note the presence of physiological patterns (spindles) only on the right hemisphere.*
C: *during IV lorazepam 1.5 mg.*
D: *5 m later: spikes and poly-spikes and suppression burst pattern on the lef hemisphere and spindles on the right.*
E: *20 m later, the girl is sleeping: important asymmetry with delta waves on the left and physiological patterns of sleep on the right.*
EMG1+EMG1 = right deltoid muscle; PNG1+PNG1 = left deltoid muscle; MKR+MKR = not used.

variable posture during the seizure (extension of one limb and flexion of another). It is mainly the sampling of several muscles on both sides of the body which permits the analysis of clinical events. In one typical example, onset occurred in the face with opening of the eyes preceding the motor phenomena, with deviation of the eyeballs, head and mouth. The patient seemed to be unresponsive and did not react to stimuli. Clonic jerks started in the face before involving the limbs. They were asynchronous, with an asymmetric frequency (vibratory on one side and slower in the other) and stopped on one side and persisted on the other. They lasted from 30 seconds to two minutes. The autonomic symptoms were slight and occurred only at the end of the longest attacks: cyanosis, apnoea, hypersalivation and respiratory obstruction.

The EEG discharge is always bilateral but may vary. Bilateral abnormalities may occur from onset as a slow spike or SW, sometimes followed by a brief attenuation, then rapid activity and slow waves, still bilateral *(Figure 5)*, in contrast to the clinical events. Abnormalities may also be initially bilateral but become and remain asymmetric during the seizure. In some cases, they are bilateral but asymmetric at the very onset. The postictal EEG shows either a diffuse flattening or a diffuse slowing. Sometimes, the end of the seizure is not easy to recognize and the child continues sleeping. This asymmetry recorded in EEGs during the GTCS has been also described by Kanazawa (1992) and Ogino (1986).

"Unstable seizures" (recorded in 11 cases). These are characterised by the topographic changes of the ictal EEG discharge in the same seizure. The clinical manifestations are similar to those of the "falsely generalised" seizures with asymmetric and asynchronous tonic and clonic movements, sometimes predominant on one side or shifting from one side to the other. However, the EEG discharge involves different parts of the brain, without any regularity. It can start in a localised area of one hemisphere then spread to the whole hemisphere of origin, or to a different area of the same hemisphere, or to a discrete area of the contralateral hemisphere, or asymmetrically to both hemispheres, and subsequently involve again the area where it originated from. The end of the discharge can occur either in this hemisphere or contralaterally *(Figure 6)*. However, the routes of propagation are very variable from one seizure to the next in the same patient, even in the same recording.

The relationship between clinical events and accompanying EEG is not always clear.

All these convulsive seizures may be prolonged (more than 30 minutes) or repeated, developing into status epilepticus which requires intravenous drug administration and, often, respiratory support. The frequency of convulsive status is reported by all authors, mainly in the first years: 71% (Oguni *et al.*, 2001), 73.5% (Fontana *et al.*, 2004), 30% (Caraballo & Fejerman, 2006), and 74.2% (Akiyama *et al.*, 2010). Sometimes, they are intractable and result in patient death. In a recent Japanese survey of 623 patients (Sakauchi *et al.*, 2011), death due to acute encephalopathy with status epilepticus was recorded in 21 (3.4%).

In the vast majority of the cases, these episodes of status are not followed by neurological sequelæ. However, recently, seven cases with such sequelæ were reported, including severe residual neurological deficits (Oguni *et al.*, 2001), hemiconvulsion-hemiplegia syndrome (Caraballo & Fejerman, 2006; Sakakibara *et al.*, 2009), and severe cognitive and neurological deterioration (Chipaux *et al.*, 2010). In the latter cases, the authors discussed the possible role of high doses of barbiturates. Sato *et al.* (1995) reported one patient who developed rhabdomyolysis during two episodes of febrile convulsive status epilepticus, with a complete recovery in spite of renal failure and liver dysfunction.

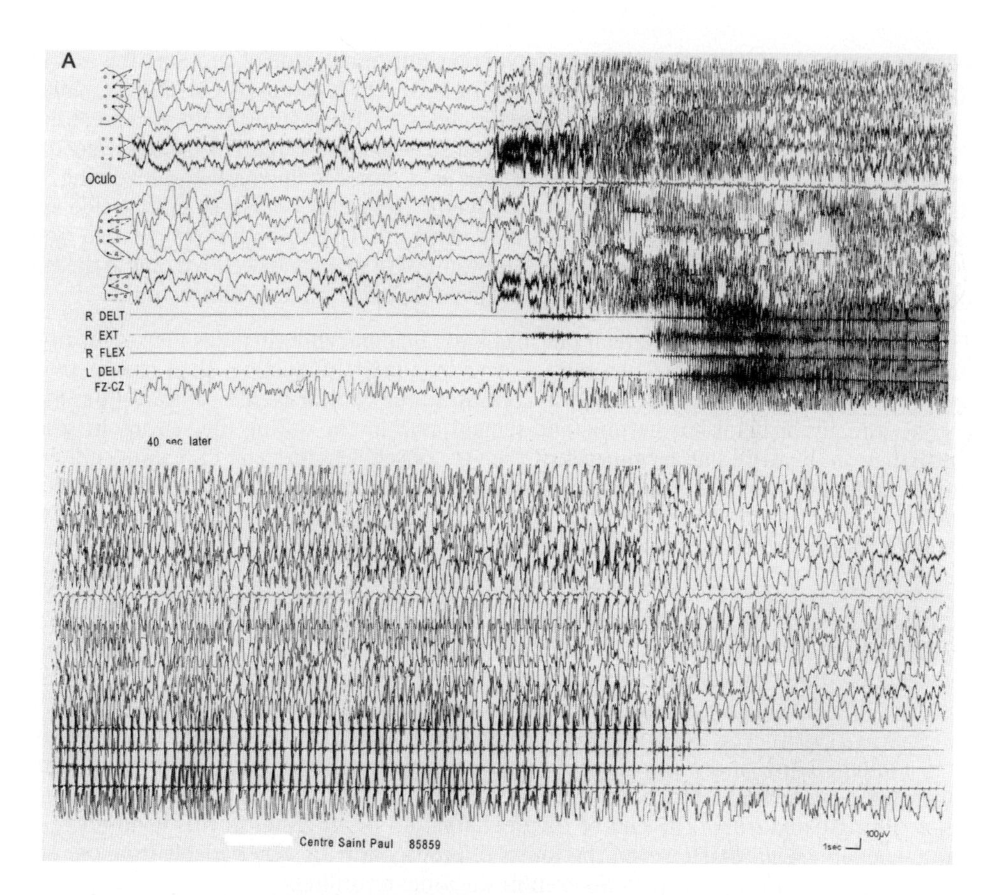

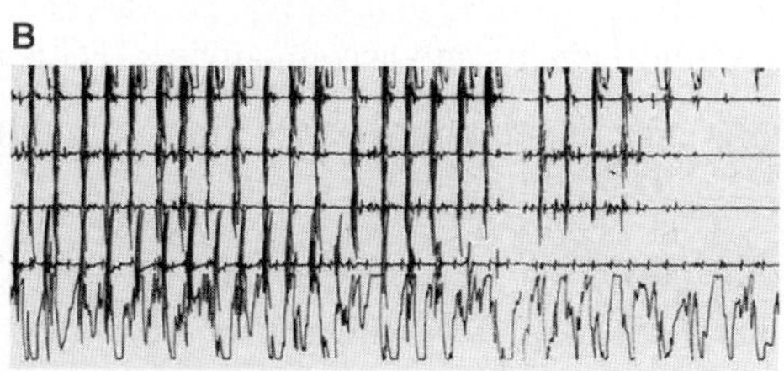

Figure 5a and b. *"Falsely generalised" seizure in a five-year, six-month-old boy.*
5a: *Top: at onset a generalized slow spike followed by a low voltage theta activity, then bilateral fast activity of higher voltage over the left hemisphere. Note on the EMG recording that a slight bilateral tonic contraction begins 2 s after the EEG onset, remits, then is followed by an irregular tonic contraction associated with a vibratory aspect. Bottom: 40 s later: diffuse spikes and waves associated with bilateral myoclonias which become progressively asynchronous (see the enlargement of the EMG polygraphy in* ***5b****) and stop on the left deltoid before they stop on the right muscles. At the end of the seizure note the absence of a flattening but the presence of high-voltage delta waves.*
R DELT = right deltoid muscle; R EXT = right wrist extensor muscle; R FLEX = right wrist flexor muscle; L DELT = left deltoid muscle; oculo = oculogramme.

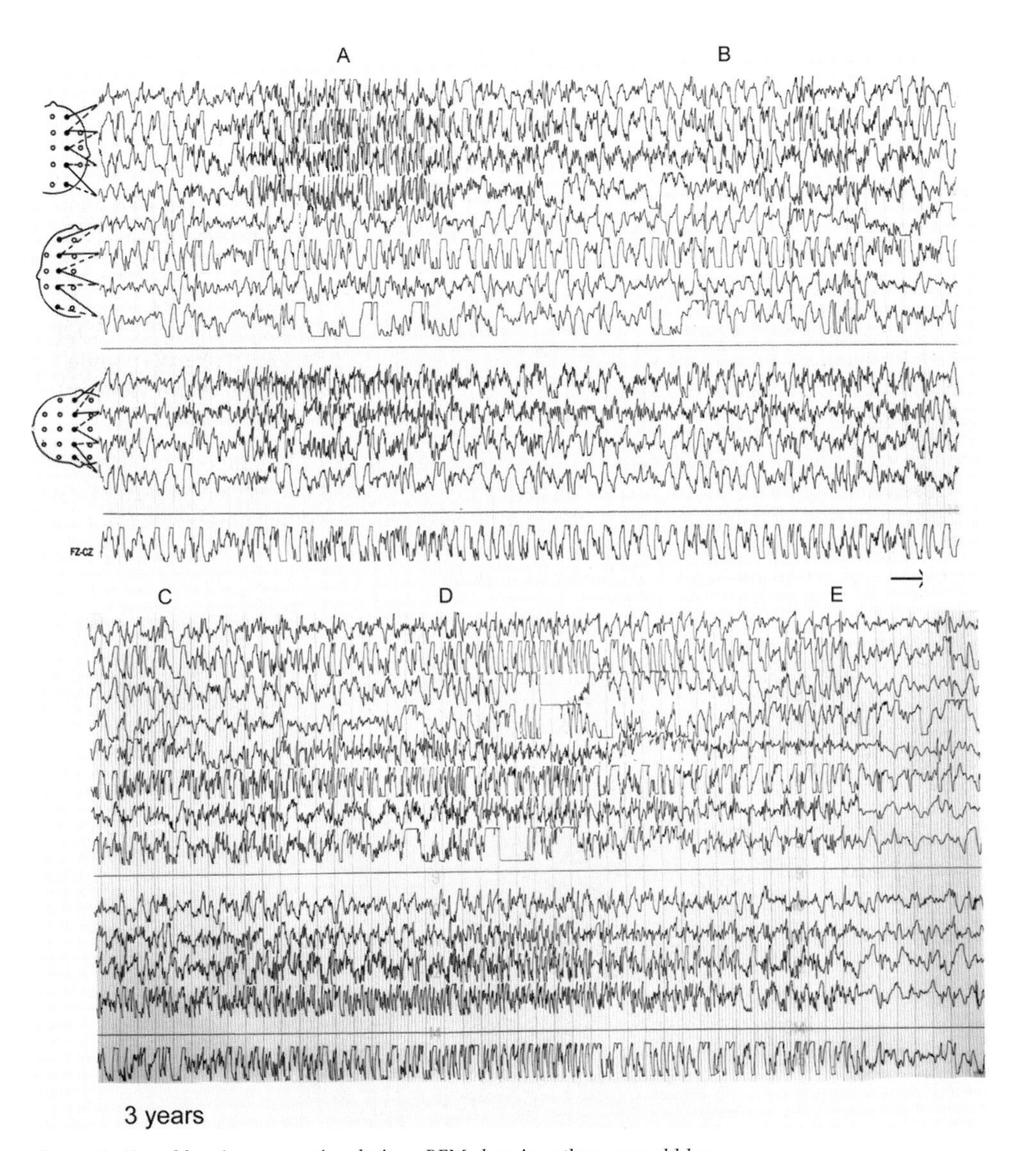

Figure 6. *Unstable seizure occurring during nREM sleep in a three-year-old boy.*
Top: *brief diffuse lowering of voltage intermixed with fast activity on the right hemisphere, then spikes and slow waves evident only on the right hemisphere during 10 s, followed by a more or less rhythmic activity around 10 Hz on the right centro-parietal area. 20 s after the onset of that activity a similar activity appears on the left fronto-centro-temporal region.*
Bottom: *continuation of the seizure: the activity is progressively associated with slow waves on the left hemisphere, becoming slower at the end of the seizure.*
A) cough, B) nothing noted, C) slight diffuse tremor, D) deviation of eyes and head to the right, E) no deficit.

Myoclonic seizures

We distinguish between ictal and interictal myoclonia. Ictal myoclonia are concomitant with a paroxysmal discharge on the EEG, whereas interictal myoclonia do not have an EEG correlate. The latter will be considered in a subsequent chapter.

Myoclonic seizures appear between the ages of one and five years, sometimes earlier, with an average of one year and five months (Caraballo & Fejerman, 2006), one year and eight months (Dravet *et al.*, 2005a, b), 18 ± 14 months (Oguni *et al.*, 2001), and two years and two months (Ohki *et al.*, 1997). They are difficult to analyze due to their variability.

Myoclonic seizures can be massive, involving the whole body, particularly axial muscles, leading to hurling of objects held by the child and falling. However, the intensity of seizures is variable, and they are sometimes barely discernible. When they are attenuated, they can involve only the axial muscles (head and trunk), causing a small movement forwards or backwards.

Some parents describe sudden falls to the ground without apparent myoclonic jerks and several authors reported atonic seizures which were never recorded by polygraphy. We did not observe or record such drop attacks. We only recorded an atonic component associated with myoclonia during a head drop *(Figure 7)*. Thus, purely atonic seizures leading to drop attacks in this syndrome remain to be documented.

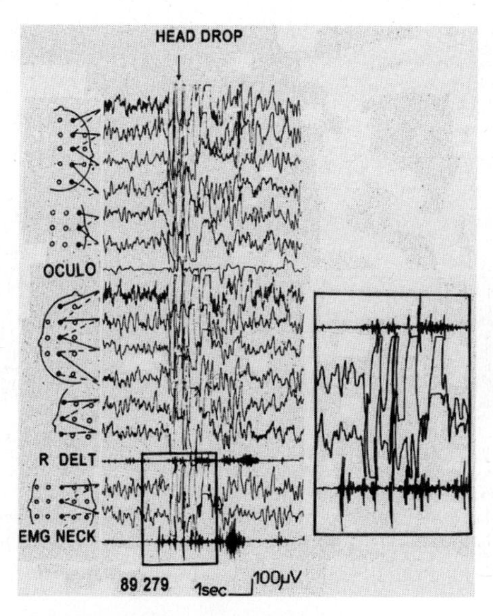

Figure 7. *Myoclonic-atonic seizure in a two-year, seven-month-old boy.*
One discharge of rapid, high voltage, generalized spikes and waves, during 1 s, accompanied by a brief head drop. On the right, the enlargement of the image shows the postmyoclonic atonia responsible for the clinical event.
R DELT = right deltoid muscle; oculo = oculogramme.

Myoclonic seizures can be either isolated or grouped in brief bursts, consisting of two or three jerks. They are very frequent, occurring several times a day, sometimes incessantly. In some children they are observed only on awakening or in the minutes or hours preceding a seizure. They persist during drowsiness and disappear during slow sleep. They can be initiated by photic stimulation, variation in light intensity, closure of the eyes or fixation on patterns. They do not seem to be accompanied by changes in consciousness, except when they occur at very close intervals.

The polygraphic EEG recordings demonstrate that myoclonic seizures are accompanied by generalised SWs or multiple SWs, at 3 Hz or faster, with higher voltage in fronto-central areas and the vertex *(Figure 8)*. Their duration is usually brief (one to three seconds) but can sometimes be longer (up to 10 seconds). The EMG can show post-myoclonic inhibition corresponding to the head drop. According to Guerrini *et al.* (2005a) who performed a neurophysiological study of these myoclonic jerks using back averaging, the generalised jerks appeared to be caused by the spread of cortical activity which originated independently from multiple cortical areas.

These discharges can be similar to those observed in benign myoclonic epilepsy of infancy even if, as documented by Hirano *et al.* (2009), jerks are predominantly characterised by extensor postural changes of the trunk and upper limbs.

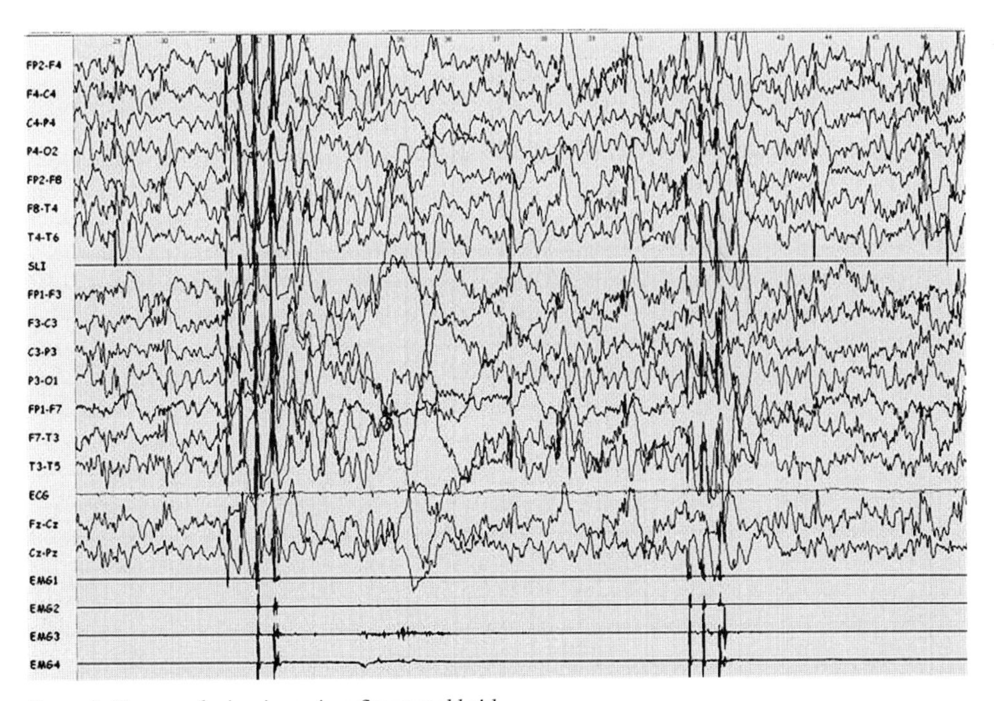

Figure 8. *Two myoclonic seizures in a five-year-old girl.*
Awake EEG: 2 bursts of generalized spikes and waves accompanied by generalized jerks, and independent multifocal spikes over the fronto-central and parieto-occipital areas.
EMG1 = right deltoid muscle; EMG2 = left deiltoid muscle; EMG3 = right wrist extensor muscle; EMG4 = right wrist flexor muscle; ECG = electrocardiogramme.

In our series, the occurrence of myoclonic status was rare *(Figure 9)*, but in many cases the recurrence in clusters could culminate into a convulsive seizure. Other authors also describe these episodes of status in their patients, sometimes lasting more than one day (Dalla Bernardina *et al.*, 1987; Yakoub *et al.*, 1992).

Atypical absence seizures

These can appear at different ages, either between one and three years, together with myoclonic attacks, or later on, from five to 12 years. In the series of Ohki *et al.* (1997), they occurred between four months and six years of age. They are divided into atypical absence seizures with unresponsiveness only, or with a more or less obvious myoclonic component. Their duration varies from three to 10 seconds. In the former type, eyelid myoclonia and head fall can be observed. In the latter type, when the myoclonic component is pronounced, it is difficult to differentiate these atypical absences from myoclonic attacks.

In fact, both are probably the expression of the same epileptic process with different intensity and duration. Their frequency is variable in the different series (from 40 to 93%). This variability can be explained by two factors: an overlap with the myoclonic seizures and diagnostic difficulties in children who have behavioural disturbances. Both seizure types correspond to generalised, irregular SWs at 2-3.5 Hz *(Figure 10)*. However, occasionally, absences with rhythmic, generalised SWs at 3 Hz, similar to those observed in childhood absence epilepsy, have been recorded (Dulac & Arthuis, 1982) *(Figure 11)*.

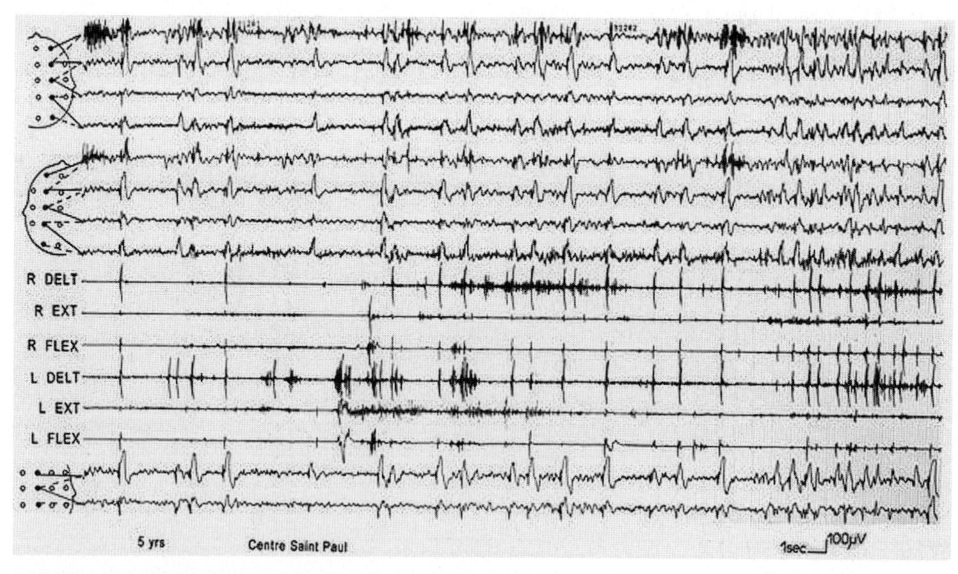

Figure 9. *Myoclonic jerk status in a five-year-old boy.*
Rapid high-voltage generalized fast spikes and waves accompanied by myoclonic jerks more important on the deltoid muscles, sometimes associated with a tonic contraction.
R DELT = right deltoid muscle; R EXT = right wrist extensor muscle; R FLEX = right wrist flexor muscle; L DELT = left deltoid muscle; L EXT = left wrist extensor muscle; L FLEX = left wrist flexor muscle.

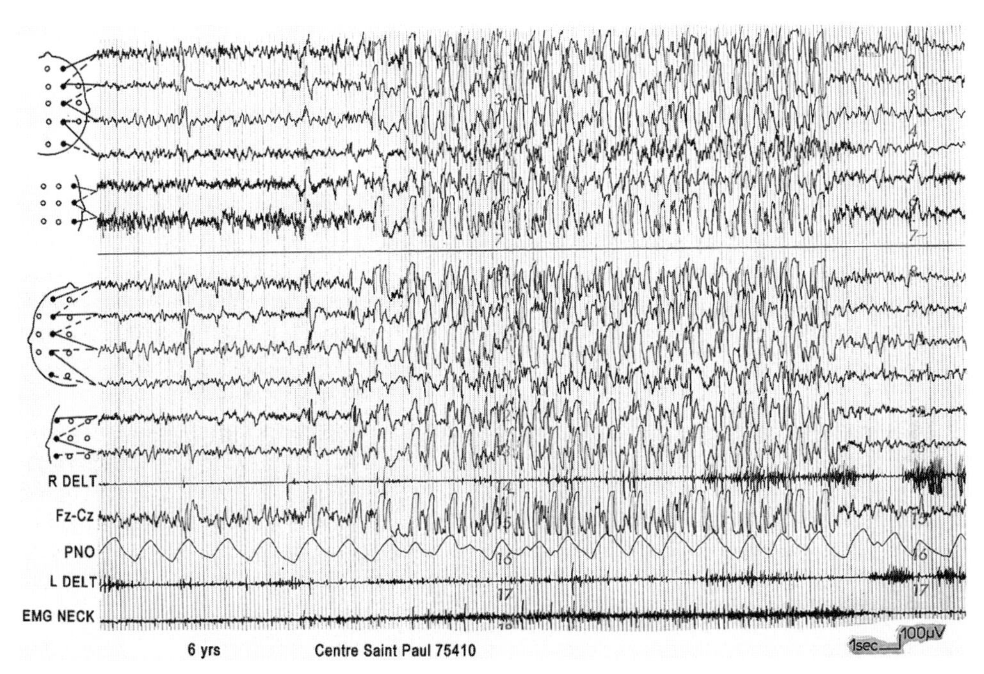

Figure 10. *Atypical absence in a six-year-old girl.*
Discharge of irregular, high voltage, diffuse spikes and waves accompanied by arhythmic, slight myoclonic jerks, visible on the left deltoid and the EMG neck, and a change in the respiration.
R DELT = right deltoid muscle; L DELT = left deltoid muscle; PNO = pneumogramme.

Ohmori *et al.* (2001) recorded atypical absences with either predominance or onset of SWs in the occipital regions.

In a few subjects, absence status can be observed (Bureau & Dalla Bernardina, 2011). This status appears progressively as impairment of consciousness of fluctuating intensity, without motor manifestations. The EEG is characterised by subcontinuous sequences of slow poly-SWs, fluctuating in amplitude, diffuse on both hemispheres, with anterior predominance. Episodes of absence status are long-lasting, and can disappear spontaneously during sleep but reappear upon awakening if sleep duration is brief.

Obtundation status

These represent a relatively characteristic manifestation, reported in several series with a frequency of: 40% (Dalla Bernardina *et al.*, 1987), 43.5% (Oguni *et al.*, 2001), 43% (Fontana *et al.*, 2004), and 30% (Dravet *et al.*, 2005a, b). However, they were not reported in three series (Ohki *et al.*, 1997; Caraballo & Fejerman, 2006; Ragona *et al.*, 2010). We recorded 18 episodes of obtundation status in 11 patients, between two years and four months and 19 years and nine months (mean: eight years and eight months) (Bureau & Dalla Bernardina, 2011).

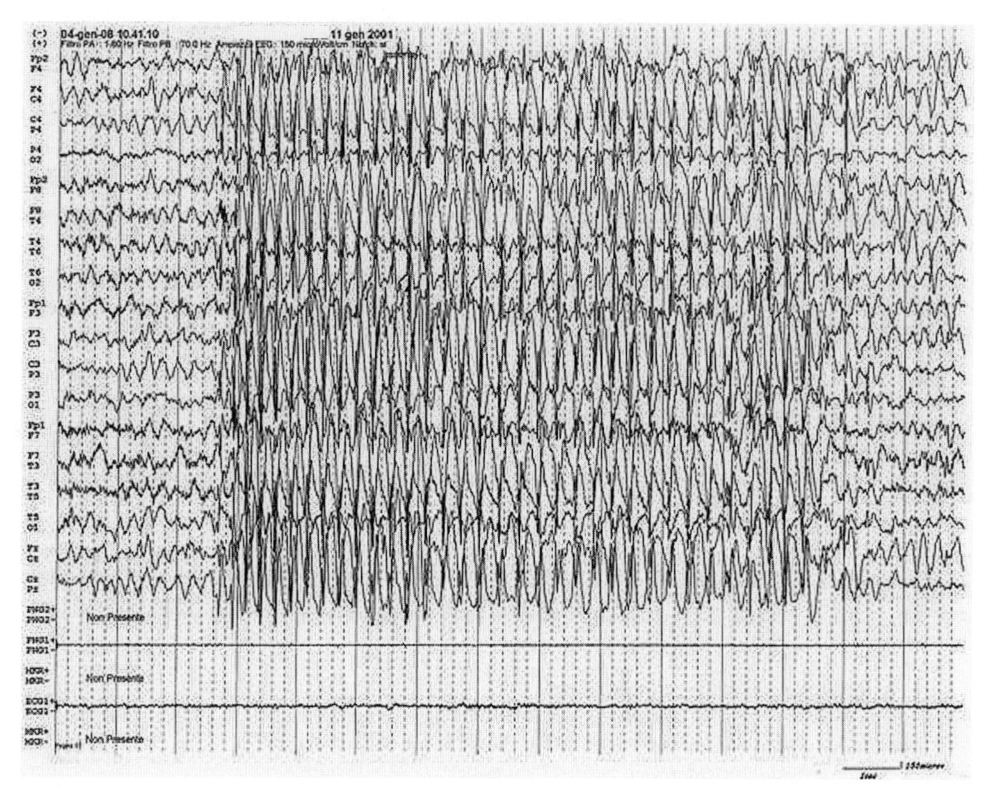

Figure 11. *Atypical absence in an eight-year-old boy.*
Discharge of regular, high voltage, generalized spikes and waves at 3 Hz, very similar to the discharge observed in the absences of Chilhood Absence Epilepsy. Clinically, no obvious event was observed during this absence, but a subtle change in the mimics.
NB: 1 cm = 100 microvolts.

Obtundation status consists of an impairment of consciousness, variable in intensity, with fragmentary and segmental, erratic myoclonia, of low amplitude, involving the limbs and face, sometimes associated with drooling and a slight increase of muscle tone. Random recurrent massive jerks are intercalated. According to their degree of consciousness, patients may or may not react to stimuli or perform simple activities (*e.g.* manipulate toys, eat), interrupted by short episodes of complete unresponsiveness and staring. Strong sensory stimulations can interrupt the status but never definitively. In four of our patients, myoclonia built up into brief synchronous fits. Convulsive seizures could either occur at the onset, during or at the end of status. These periods could be prolonged for several hours, even several days, and maintained by environmental light stimuli, eye closure or pattern fixation (for two recorded episodes of status, this included dotted lines on a wall and a TV screen, respectively). The EEG is usually characterised by diffuse dysrhythmia of slow waves, intermingled with focal and diffuse spikes *(Figure 12)*, sharp waves and SWs, of higher voltage in the anterior brain and vertex regions, without temporal relationship between spikes and myoclonic jerks, except

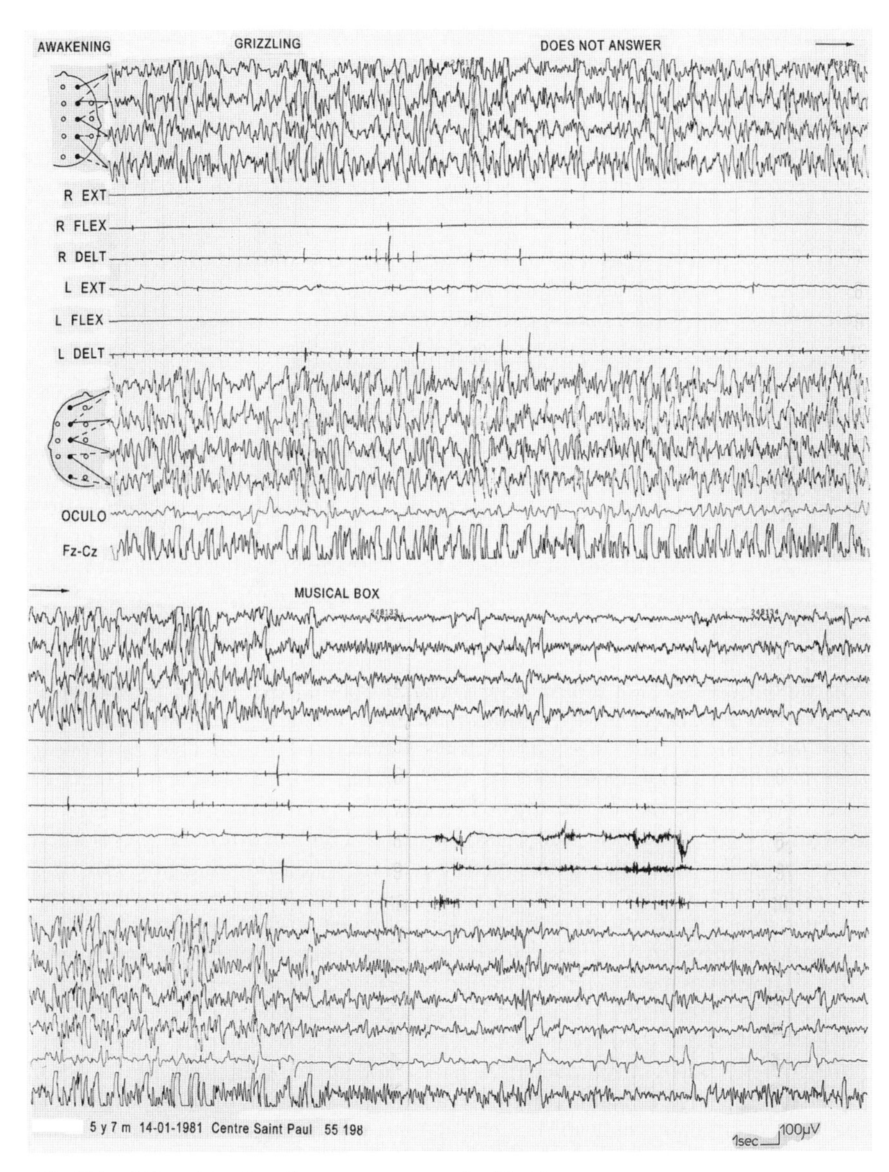

Figure 12. *Obtundation status in a five-year, seven-month-old girl.*
Top: The EEG shows slow waves intermixed with spikes and fast activities. Clinically, impairment of consciousness with erratic, fragmentary myoclonias.
Bottom: when presented with a music box, the child, who is clearly interested, becomes very present and reaches for the toy. The EEG shows an abrupt interruption of the diffuse slow activity, with persisting isolated spikes; note the persistence of erratic myoclonias that have become less frequent and less ample.
R EXT = right wrist extensor muscle; R FLEX = right wrist flexor muscle; R DELT = right deltoid muscle; L EXT = left wrist extensor muscle; L FLEX = left wrist flexor muscle; L DELT = left deltoid muscle; Oculo = oculogramme.

during the myoclonic fits. This characteristic picture was also described by Ohmori *et al.* (2001). We never recorded rhythmic SWs as observed in generalised absence status. Intravenous or rectal diazepam attenuated but did not stop this status which we classified now rather as non convulsive status than as atypical absence status. In the four patients reported by Yasuda *et al.* (1989), this status always occurred after a GTCS, lasted from seven to 16 minutes, and was accompanied by diffuse high-voltage slow waves, occasionally notched by small spikes in the frontal regions.

Other EEG aspects were described by Oguni *et al.* (2001): pseudorhythmic diffuse high-amplitude, irregular slow waves, gradually slowing down in frequency, and bursts of bilateral, diffuse high-voltage slow waves, occasionally notched with small spikes.

In two studies, a different type of non-convulsive status was reported. Oguni *et al.* (2001) reported a girl who remained unconscious with deviation of the eyes to one side whereas her EEG showed continuous posterior irregular slow waves or SWs. Wakai *et al.* (1996a) described a boy, aged nine months, who had a prolonged episode of staring ahead, with akinesis, decreased physical tone, occasional deviation of the eyes to the right and unresponsiveness, accompanied by irregular SW complexes over the left hemisphere, predominantly in the occipito-temporal area. This condition lasted for six hours in spite of administration of antiepileptic drugs. In the second patient, the ictal EEG was similar to that observed for unilateral seizures. These two cases of status were diagnosed as *complex partial status* by the authors.

Focal seizures

Simple partial seizures (SPS) of motor type or complex partial seizures (CPS), with prominent autonomic symptoms, occur in 43-78.6% of patients in the largest series (Oguni *et al.*, 2001; Ohmori *et al.*, 2001; Caraballo & Fejerman, 2006; Ragona *et al.*, 2010). They can appear early, from four months to four years (Ohki *et al.*, 1997). In our series (Dravet *et al.*, 2005a, b), they were described in 32 patients (53%); four with only SPS, 17 with only CPS and 11 with both. SPS were either versive seizures or clonic jerks limited to a limb or one hemiface, or a combination of the two. CPS were characterised by unresponsiveness, autonomic phenomena (pallor, cyanosis, rubefaction, respiratory changes, drooling, and sweating), oral automatisms, hypotonia, rarely stiffness, and sometimes eyelid or distal myoclonus. When the symptomatology is mild, they are difficult to distinguish from atypical absences if the EEG is not recorded. The two partial seizure types may occur with secondary generalisation. Surprisingly, we have recorded these only in three patients, at 20 months, four years and nine months and 12 years, respectively. The first occurred upon awakening and was a CPS, with unresponsiveness, right deviation of the eyes, arrhythmic myoclonia, pallor, and lip cyanosis, occurring for one minute 45 seconds, accompanied by a left temporo-occipital EEG discharge and left postictal slowing. The other two occurred during sleep EEG. The first was apparently subclinical and involved the right and left centro-temporal area, alternatively *(Figure 13)*. The second episode was not well observed clinically, and involved the right temporo-occipital and the vertex areas.

In the literature, the reported focal seizures are usually of the complex partial type with the same characteristics we have described. Ohki *et al.* (1997) recorded 25 seizures in eight patients with variable EEG features, beginning either in the frontal (six recordings), temporal (nine recordings), or occipital (six recordings) areas. In four patients, it was not possible to determine the exact onset, and in three the onset was variable from one seizure to another. Six seizures occurred with secondary generalisation.

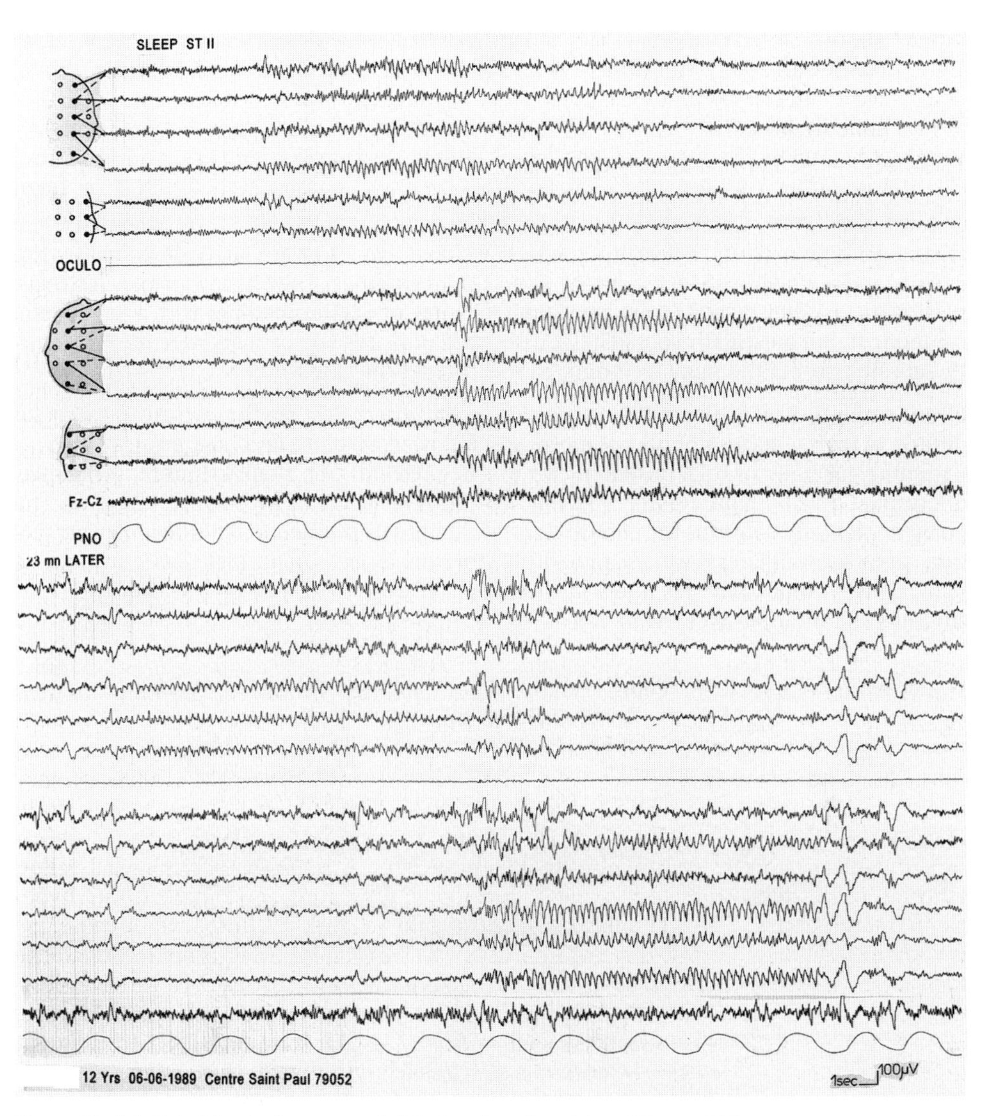

Figure 13. *Subclinical focal seizures recorded during sleep stage 2 in a 12-year-old boy.*
Top: *discharge of low voltage spikes and waves diffuse on the right hemisphere predominantly over the temporo-parietal areas. Independently, 11 s after the onset of this seizure a diffuse left spike and wave appears, followed by a discharge of low voltage spikes and waves over the left centro-temporal region.*
Bottom: *two other independent subclinical seizures on the right posterior area and on the left centrotemporal area.*
Oculo = oculogramme; PNO = pneumogramme.

While CPS are reported by most authors, SPS are reported only by some (Giovanardi-Rossi *et al.*, 1991; Yakoub *et al.*, 1992; Wang *et al.*, 1996; Sarisjulis *et al.*, 2000; Caraballo & Fejerman, 2006).

Tonic seizures

These seizures are unusual for this syndrome and such cases are mentioned in just six reports in the literature (Dulac & Arthuis, 1982; Dravet *et al.*, 1992a; Lambarri San Martin *et al.*, 1997; Ohmori *et al.*, 2001, Caraballo & Fejerman, 2006; Nabbout *et al.*, 2008). We recorded tonic seizures in nine patients, between six and 25 years of age. They are rarely described by the parents and are mainly detected during sleep EEG recordings. They have variable electroclinical features. They resemble the axial tonic seizures of LGS, sometimes with a myoclonic component, but are usually sporadic (six cases) and only in a few patients were they frequently repeated during the same recording, as it is instead the case for LGS.

In our patients, ictal EEG exhibited several aspects; either a fast rhythm which was directly diffuse, of high voltage, stopping abruptly and followed by slight and brief postictal signs, a flattening generally of brief duration (two to three seconds), or a rapid rhythm, sometimes interrupted by a flattening *(Figure 14)*, followed by slow waves or irregular diffuse SWs. The polygraphic study confirms the clinical signs; if the initial contraction is a true tonic contraction, some seconds later it can change with a vibratory aspect, intermingled with myoclonic jerks. Only in four cases was interictal sleep EEG analogous to that in LGS showing rapid rhythms and multiple SWs *(Figure 15)*.

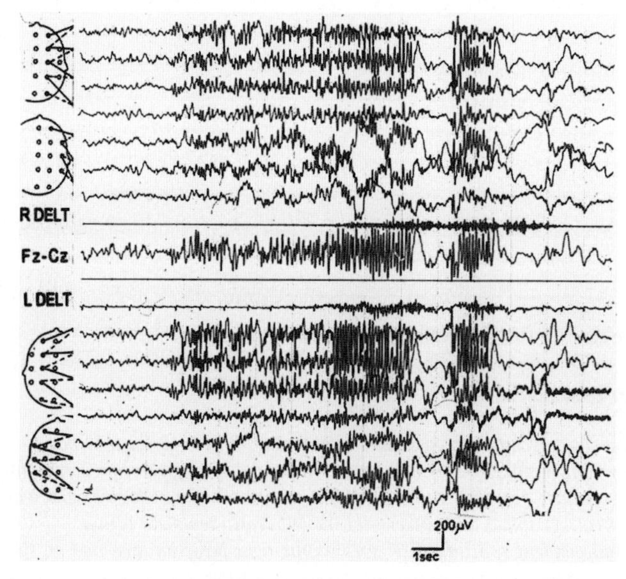

Figure 14. *Tonic seizure occurring during stage 2 sleep in an 11-year, seven-month-old girl.*
Fast rhythms increasing in voltage, more evident over the vertex and the frontal areas, predominantly on the left. 10 s after the onset, note a flattening followed by a burst of fast rhythms and a slowness of the activity. On the EMG recording (2 deltoids) tonic contraction beginning 6 s after the onset of the seizure.
R DELT = right deltoid muscle; L DELT = left deltoid muscle.

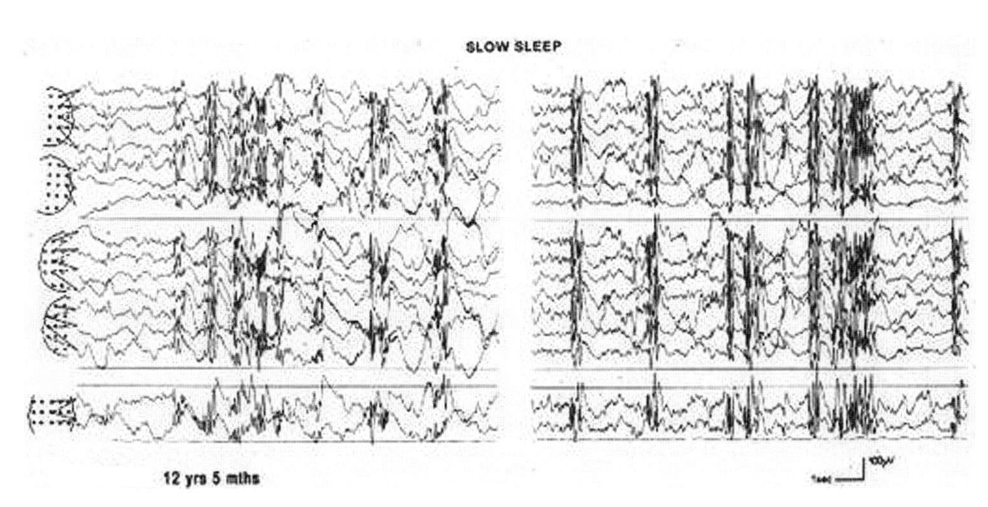

Figure 15. *Interictal sleep abnormalities in the same girl as in figure 14.*
Diffuse spikes and poly-spike-waves and bursts of fast rhythms mimicking the nREM sleep in the Lennox-Gastaut syndrome.

In a recent study, Nabbout *et al.*, (2008) recorded tonic seizures in five patients and described an interictal EEG pattern consisting of frontal, slow double or triple spikes followed or not by slow waves while awake and activated by sleep, which is unusual in patients with DS.

Other paroxysmal events are sometimes described by the parents, which may be epileptic in nature but difficult to classify.

Triggering factors

One of the main symptoms that characterises DS patients is their extremely low epileptic threshold to external, as well as internal, stimuli. This sensitivity, which is especially observed in the youngest children, is a major factor of anxiety for the parents who tend to guard their child from situations associated with seizure risk. The following conditions will be discussed: temperature variation and hot baths, light, patterns, physical exercise, excitation, and emotions. Other potential precipitating factors are noted by the parents but remain anecdotal.

Temperature variation

At the time of the discovery of this disease, we underlined the "fever sensitivity" of patients. However, it is more appropriate to speak of body temperature variation because the temperature level that can trigger a seizure is often below the level associated with fever. Indeed, fever corresponds to a body temperature equal to or higher than 37.8° C, but seizures can occur when the temperature is less than 37° C. This increase of temperature may be accompanied by an infection. Sometimes temperature increases after the end of the seizure and at other times quickly decreases and there is no recognizable reason for this small peak. Parents are aware of this sensitivity and constantly look at children and measure their temperature at the minor sign of "fever" in order to prevent a seizure.

Temperature sensitivity is also apparent when the child takes a hot bath. This was first described by Japanese authors (Ogino *et al.*, 1985) since whole body immersion in hot water (39° C to 42° C for 5-10 minutes) is a cultural occurrence in Japan. Awaya *et al.* (1989) performed an impressive study, demonstrating the crucial role of increasing temperature unrelated to infection or physical exercise. They recorded the video-EEG of seven children with SMEI in hot water immersion, and monitored their temperature continuously. Clinically overt seizures were all provoked after 7-25 minutes of hot water immersion, when rectal temperature rose above 38° C. In addition, five patients clearly showed an increase in frequency and duration of epileptic discharges with elevation of the temperature, which culminated in clinical seizures: absence seizures, GTCS, complex focal seizures, and massive myoclonic jerks. In European countries, this effect of hot baths is rare, and was reported in eight of 37 Italian patients (Ragona *et al.*, 2010).

External temperature can also represent an aggravating factor and some patients have more seizures in summer and in hot regions.

Patients clearly have an increased susceptibility to infection; infections of the upper respiratory tract are frequent and pneumonia can be severe. However, immunological studies did not show abnormalities that could explain this susceptibility (Nieto *et al.*, 2000; Oguni *et al.*, 2001).

Photosensitivity and pattern sensitivity

Photosensitivity can be manifested as a pathological response to either intermittent photic stimulation (IPS), bright light or intense contrast between bright light and darkness. The effect of eye closure can also be related to photosensitivity, as well as the effect of patterns and television, since they can produce highly contrasted stimuli. All these stimuli can provoke the different seizure types: eyelid myoclonia, atypical absences (usually with myoclonus) and clonic seizures (with or without focal onset). Pattern sensitivity is not always easy to detect in young children and should therefore be carefully looked for. All kinds of more or less contrasting patterns, present in the daily environment, can be efficacious and include: geometrical designs or dotted lines on walls, roofs, pavements, clothes, window screens, escalators, roof tiles, stony paths; letters and designs in books for children, and so on.

Photosensitivity is difficult to analyse because it does not remain constant during the course of the disease. A discrepancy between the laboratory EEG and everyday clinical photosensitivity can be observed, partly due to the use of various photic stimulators, of which some are less efficacious than others in detecting a photoparoxysmal response (Specchio *et al.*, 2011). However, since the first descriptions, photosensitivity has been reported as one of the main features (Dravet, 1978; Dravet *et al.*, 1982; Dalla Bernardina *et al.*, 1982), and although it is mentioned in most studies, it has been carefully studied in only a few.

In our 1992 series (Dravet *et al.*, 1992a), EEG photosensitivity was observed at least once in the course of the disease in 31 patients (49%), with onset between three months and five years and six months. In eight patients it persisted. In 10 it was observed only in one recording. In seven children we were able to estimate its duration: from three months to 11 years and six months. We also observed the triggering effect of eye closure (10/63) *(Figure 16)*, patterns (7/63) and television (1/63) for myoclonus and SWs. Self stimulation by eye closure or pattern fixation was observed in 10/63 patients. Eye closure may provoke episodes of "eye fluttering", consisting of subtle eyelid myoclonus and rolling-up of eyeballs, with decreased

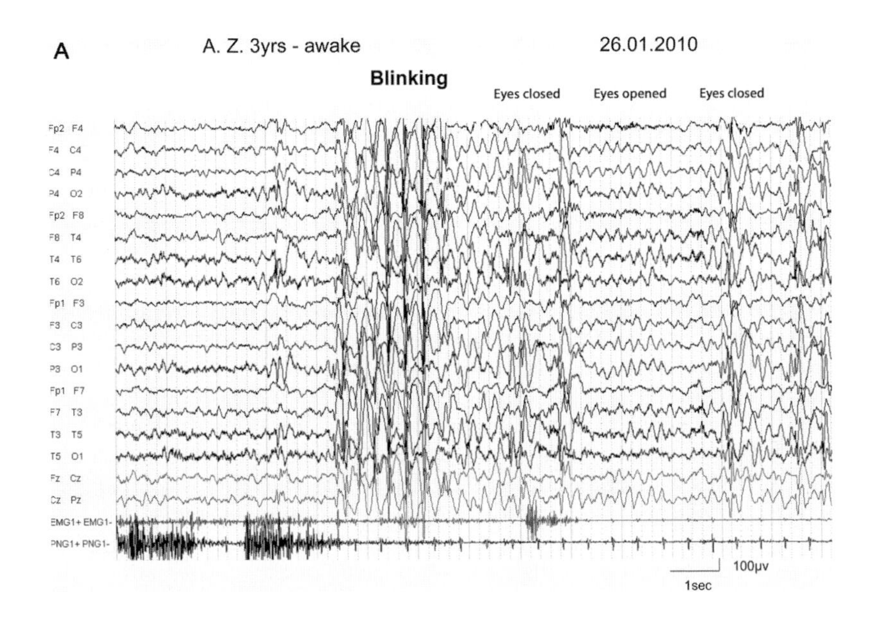

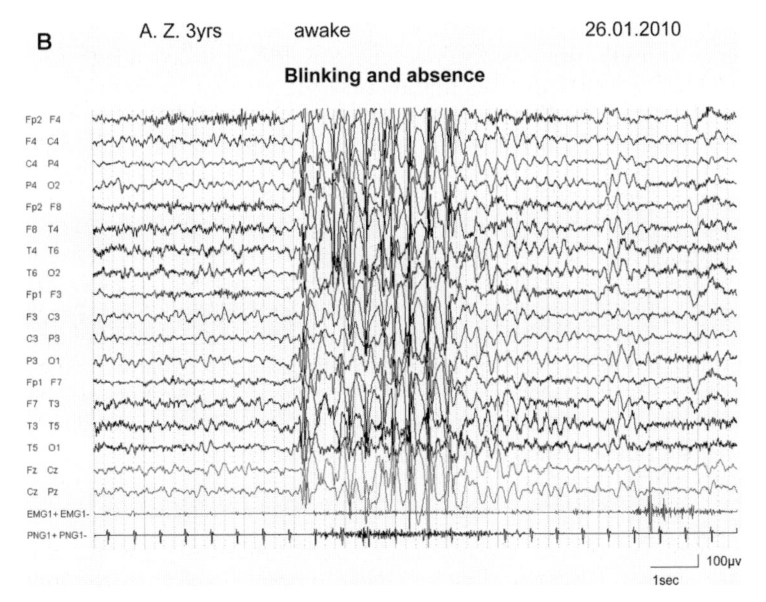

Figure 16a and b. *Eye closure effect in a three-year-old boy.*
A: *eye closure triggers a burst of diffuse, irregular spikes and waves and slow waves, associated with an eye blinking, which is interrupted by eye opening and re-appears when the child closes his eyes again.*
B: *this more regular discharge, also provoked by eye closure, is associated with a blinking and a brief loss of responsiveness*
EMG1+EMG1 = right deltoid muscle; PNG1+PNG1 = left deltoid muscle.

responsiveness. These episodes are briefly interrupted by eye opening but can last several minutes.

Ohki *et al.* (1997) also observed, over time, variability of photosensitivity in four patients. Ragona *et al.* (2010) reported a clear history of pattern sensitivity in 11/37 patients (in response to: sun on water, window screens, garments, an escalator, and roof tiles).

In their series of 53 patients, Fontana *et al.* (2004) found photosensitivity in 38%, pattern sensitivity in 17% and self stimulation in 40%.

In the Tokyo series (Oguni *et al.*, 2001), among 39 patients, six appeared to have numerous daily attacks (more than 100-200/day) which were related to the intensity of constant light illumination, *i.e.* seizures became very frequent under bright conditions, while they were remarkably reduced in the dark. A strong response to IPS was also observed, but careful examination in one case showed no specific increase to IPS at low frequency and brightness of light had more influence. Their predominant seizure types were myoclonic seizures and atypical absences with pronounced eyelid myoclonia, the latter accompanied by occasional rhythmic retropulsion of the head. They became continuous immediately after exposure to bright illumination or sunshine. Since they frequently and easily culminated into GTCS, the patients had to wear sunglasses when going outside, or remain inside. In one patient, Miyamoto *et al.* (1993) showed constant light sensitivity, gradually decreasing around the age of five years, and photo-/pattern sensitivity at age seven. Takahashi *et al.* (1999) showed that patients with SMEI have a paroxysmal response, which is different from that of patients with idiopathic generalised epilepsy since it is dependent on the quantity of light rather than wavelength. This finding may suggest that this sensitivity to constant light is at the strongest end of the photosensitive spectrum in SMEI patients. Children with sensitivity to constant light appear to be amongst the most severe cases, especially when they discover self stimulation. This finding is confirmed by Dalla Bernardina *et al.* (1987) and Fontana *et al.* (2004).

Other stimuli

Among the other precipitating stimuli observed, the most important are physical exercise, excitation and emotions. Many parents underline the occurrence of seizures after playing in a garden, running, jumping, receiving a gift, following a reproach, participating in a celebration (Christmas, birthday, or school event), following the replacement of a teacher, *etc*, however, no relevant study has so far been published. Other anecdotal situations are reported by parents but remain isolated, such as swinging, water, and noise.

Interictal EEG

• While awake, the EEG background activity remains normal or slightly abnormal in 50% of cases. In the remaining cases, background activity becomes slow and poorly organised. In fact, background activity varies depending on the time when the EEG is performed; it is slower during periods of multiple seizures, and can be influenced by pharmacological treatments. The peculiar theta activity in fronto-central areas, already observed at onset in some patients, appears in most cases and persists throughout follow-up (Ohki *et al.*, 1997; Bureau & Dalla-Bernardina, 2011). In some cases, there are no epileptiform abnormalities. When present, they are focal and multifocal, in fronto-central or centro-temporal areas and vertex in the majority of cases, but sometimes they are prominent over the posterior areas, associated with generalised abnormalities *(Figure 17)*. There is no relationship between the site of interictal anomaly and the site of seizure origin. Abnormalities are represented by spikes, spikes and waves and poly-SWs. The generalised SW discharges are more numerous when the myoclonic fits are frequent.

Eye closure elicits subclinical or clinical discharges of spikes and SWs in 25% of the cases.

Strong photosensitivity persists in a large proportion of cases, with or without associated clinical events. In other cases there is a fluctuation of photosensitivity.

• The sleep EEG is usually well structured with physiological patterns and cyclic organisation, except when several seizures occur during the night. However, even in these cases, non-REM and REM sleep can usually be identified. The paroxysmal, generalised, as well as localised, activities are enhanced or become apparent. In four of 60 cases (in our series), the interictal EEG showed fast rhythms sometimes followed by a flattening and poly-SWs, very similar to those observed in LGS. In some cases, there is an important activation of the focal abnormalities particularly over the frontal regions, bilaterally or predominantly, in one hemisphere. These abnormalities can become continuous or subcontinuous during slow sleep and decrease during REM sleep *(Figure 18)*.

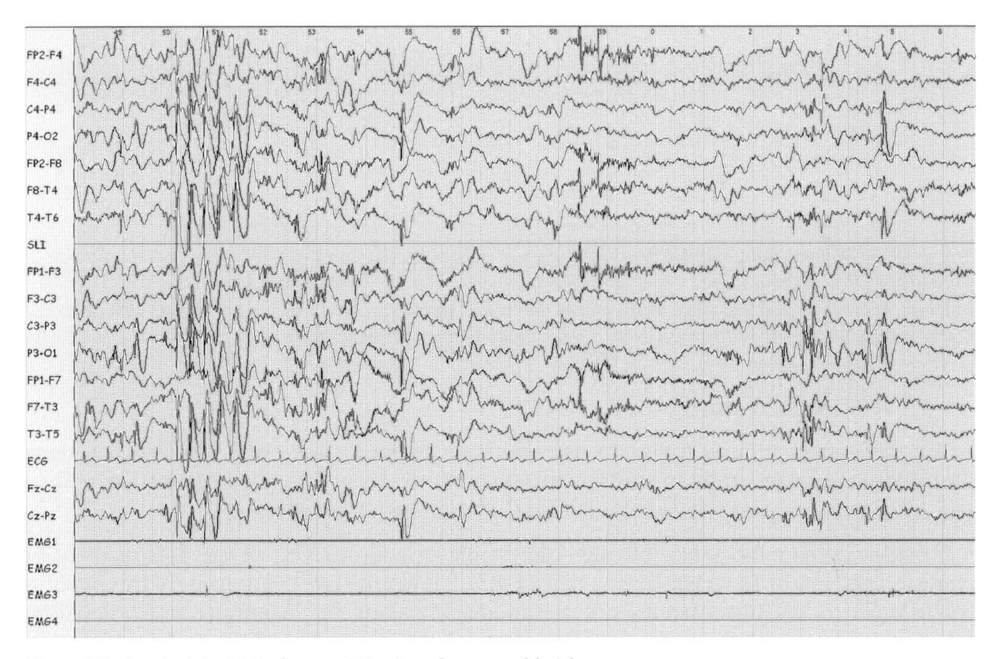

Figure 17. *Awake interictal abnormalities in a five-year-old girl.*
Awake EEG: generalized spikes and waves and independent multifocal spikes over the fronto-central and parieto-occipital areas.
EMG1 = right deltoid muscle; EMG2 = left deltoid muscle; EMG3 = right wrist extensor muscle; EMG4 = right wrist flexor muscle; ECG = electrocardiogramme.

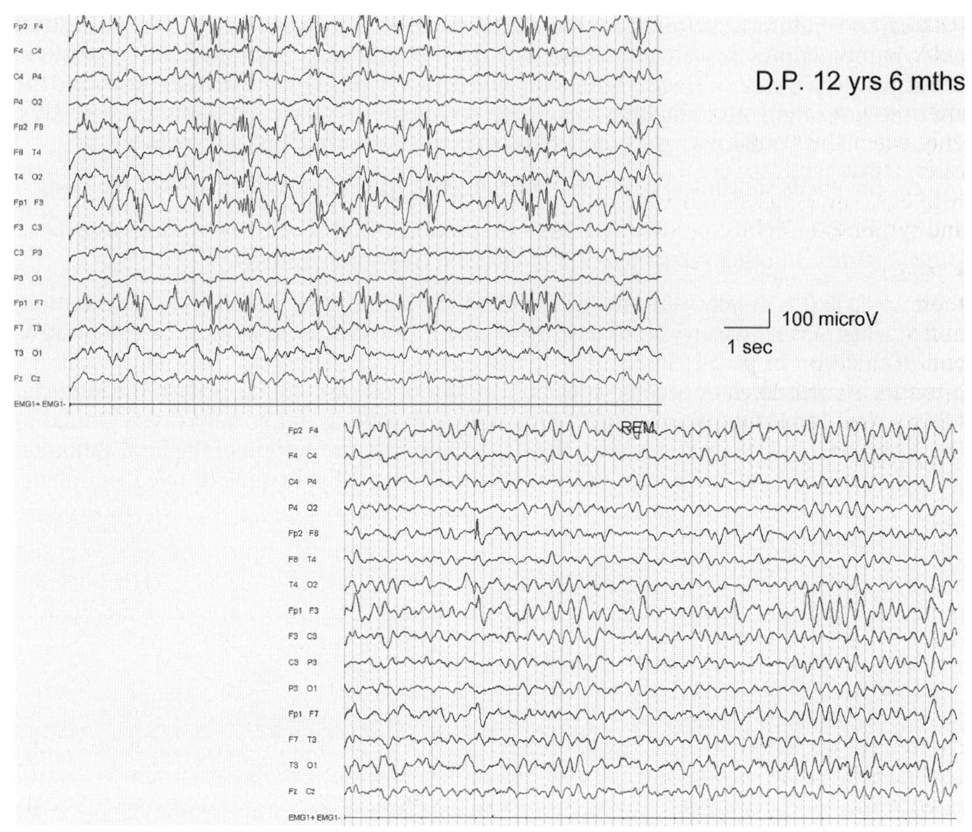

Figure 18. *Sleep interictal abnormalities during sleep in a 12-year, six-month-old girl.*
Top: *nREM sleep: subcontinuous spikes and spike and waves over the frontal areas.*
Bottom: *REM sleep: disappearance of the spikes and waves discharges, and existence of diffuse slow waves of higher voltage on the left hemisphere. Note a right fronto-temporal isolated spike.*

Neurological signs

At the very onset, infants appear to have normal developmental skills. Neurological signs progressively appear, simultaneously with psychomotor delay, but not in all patients. They consist of hypotonia, ataxia, pyramidal signs, and interictal myoclonus.

• *Hypotonia* is the most precocious sign, detectable around one year of age. It is reported in almost all patients by Dalla Bernardina *et al.* (1982). It is worthwhile being aware of this hypotonia in order to carefully examine affected toddlers, looking for hypotonia which could be responsible for further orthopaedic problems. In our practice, we advise the parents and referring doctors to pay much attention to orthopedic feet problems and prescribe early physiotherapy.

• *Ataxia* appears when the patients start to walk, usually at normal age (12-18 months). Initially, there seems to be only a delay in walking, but gait remains unsteady, stance is wide based and movements are poorly coordinated. Ataxia was reported in 83% of our first 42 cases

(Dravet *et al.*, 1985) and 80% of the first 20 cases by Dalla Bernardina *et al.* (1982). In later publications, the frequency of ataxia was reported to be variable; between 50 and 83%. Ataxia is not always obvious in the early course of epilepsy but may appear during childhood, often after status epilepticus or worsening of seizures. Some parents observe walking disturbances only when their child goes to kindergarten, in comparison with their playmates. In these cases, ataxia tends to increase with age. Conversely, in other patients, ataxia may attenuate with age. The association between hypotonia and ataxia leads to a peculiar form of walking and running, as if the children have "spaghetti legs", as described by one mother.

• *Pyramidal signs* were found in 50% of our initial patients (Dravet *et al.*, 1985) and 80% of those of Dalla Bernadina *et al.* (1982). They consist of increased deep tendon reflexes, prominent at the lower limbs, with Babinski sign. Often the children walk on tiptoes. These signs tend to increase in periods with repeated convulsive seizures and decrease when interictal intervals become longer. It is maybe for this reason that they are rarely mentioned in the other series. Caraballo & Fejerman (2006) reported them in 22.6% of their cases.

• *Interictal myoclonus.* If not constant, multifocal myoclonic jerks are frequent, appearing at the same time as the myoclonic seizures, between the age of one and five years. They are also observed in many patients who do not have myoclonic seizures They involve either the limbs, with a distal predominance, or facial muscles, independently. They are present at rest and are increased by voluntary movement. There is no concomitant change in EEG. They are more frequent during the periods of seizure exacerbation, particularly in older children with frequent nocturnal convulsive seizures, in the day after awakening from attacks.

The frequency of interictal myoclonus is variable in the different series; from 100% (Giovanardi Rossi *et al.*, 1991; Nabbout *et al.*, 2003) to 80% (Dalla Bernardina *et al.*, 1982), 33.3% (Fontana *et al.*, 2004), and 36% (Oguni *et al.*, 2001). This discrepancy is explained by two factors. First, some authors selected only the patients with myoclonic seizures, who all had interictal myoclonus. Second, interictal jerks can be difficult to single out. In some patients they are rare, sometimes appearing only before a convulsive seizure, and their recognition requires special attention. The best method of study is the polygraphic EEG recording. In a hyperactive child, they may be more obvious by asking the child to perform a precise activity such as drinking, piling up cubes, or holding a spoon. In the Marseille series of 60 patients selected on the basis of seizures recorded by video-polygraphic EEG, 51 had interictal myoclonus (85%), whereas in another series with a subset of the patients who did not benefit from a polygraphic recording, the figure was only 36% (Dravet *et al.*, 1992a).

Neurological signs are inconstantly observed during the course of the disease and modification over time is discussed in the chapter addressing long-term outcome.

• *Autonomic symptoms.* In the USA, the attention of parents and doctors has been drawn to other symptoms related to the autonomic system. An interesting study was reported by Wical *et al.* (2009) who performed a survey in a paediatric neurology clinic based on parental reports of signs reflecting autonomic dysfunction: cold extremities, red or bluish colour of the extremities, alterations in sweating, large pupils, slow emptying of the stomach, episodes of tachycardia, facial and chest flushing without identifiable cause, and clusters of at least four of the signs occurring together for at least 15 minutes. Frequency was reported as "never" or "very rarely", "monthly", "weekly", "several times per week" or "daily". This questionnaire was offered to parents of patients with DS (54) and parents of patients with other neurological diagnoses, excluding cerebral palsy, severe neurological impairment or neurodegenerative disorders, matched for other criteria (78). The mean number of dysautonomic events occurring at least weekly was 2.89 in the DS group *vs* 0.65 in the comparison group ($p = 0.001$). Knowing that topiramate (TPM) can decrease sweating, all children on TPM were withdrawn from both groups, the difference remaining significant: 2.65 in the DS group *vs* 0.56 in the comparison group ($p = 0.001$). In spite of its retrospective nature, this survey seems to show that autonomic dysfunction is common in children with DS. This finding deserves to be studied in more detail as it might be related to the increased risk of SUDEP in these patients.

3. Psychomotor and Cognitive Development

Developmental delay becomes progressively evident from the second year on. Usually, children start walking at normal age but an unsteady gait develops for an unusually long time. Sometimes, after the first independent steps, the child falls because he/she has a seizure, becomes afraid and does not dare to start walking again unsupported for some weeks.

Language also starts at normal age, with lalation and babble in the first year, but progresses very slowly and many patients do not reach the stage of constructing elementary sentences.

Fine motor abilities do not develop well and patients are disturbed by myoclonus and lack of good hand-eye coordination, which prevents them from acquiring the ability to carry out daily activities and play. Most children cannot draw a picture and, later on, only manage to write in capital letters.

Poor attention is one of the major factors responsible for their learning disabilities. Other factors are hyperactive and recalcitrant behaviour and stubbornness. They are often restless, do not listen to adults, and are not interested in playing with educative toys and participating in the usual activities associated with their age. Conversely, they may be able to do puzzles and watch cartoons repetitively.

Reports of speech- and physio-therapy, and examples of drawings at different ages are shown in the *Annexes 1 and 2.*

Older Psychometric Data

Several authors have reported psychometric data.

- *Dalla Bernardina et al. (1987)* categorised 29 subjects, followed until a mean age of 11 years and eight months, into three groups: nine subjects had average speech but low scholastic level (poor prognosis); nine spoke only with isolated words and were delayed in school (poorer prognosis); and 11 lacked speech and did not attend school (the poorest prognosis). The factors that seemed to negatively influence this cognitive evolution were the presence of myoclonus (myoclonic status, massive jerks, and interictal myoclonus), generalised/unilateral clonic seizures, self-stimulation, absence status, and visual sensitivity.

• *Giovanardi-Rossi et al. (1991)* reported less severe impairment in 15 patients with a mean age of 14.5 years. Mental retardation was present in all cases, being severe in 11 (Intelligence Quotient [IQ] lower than 50), and moderate in four (IQ between 50 and 75). Language was structured in all cases, but expression and content were poor and below range values for the age group. Behavioural and/or affective disorders were present in 11 patients and included: hyperactivity (seven cases), aggressiveness (four cases), opposition (six cases), fatuousness (two cases), and affective relational disorders (four cases).

• *Yakoub et al. (1992)* reported 20 patients, of whom three were without myoclonic syndrome, followed until a mean age of six years and two months. All patients had behavioural disorders and speech delay. Twelve underwent psychometric evaluation with the Brunet-Lézine test, at a mean age of five years; the developmental quotient (DQ) was around 50 in five cases, around 60 in three, and around 70 in four. In two patients, the DQ measurement was repeated and was over 80 at 18 and 21 months, and only 70 at five years, respectively.

• *Fujiwara et al. (1992)* studied 29 patients, with either typical SMEI, atypical SMEI, or intractable epilepsy with GTCS in childhood, followed for at least five years (range: six years and seven months to 20 years, median: 10 years and 11 months). All patients presented with poor development and moderate to severe mental retardation.

• *Wang et al. (1996)* reported 10 patients followed until the mean age of four years and one month. All had developmental speech delay with disturbances in articulation and verbal production, hyperactivity, attention deficit and clumsiness. Intelligence was assessed in five patients aged more than four years and all revealed IQ scores between 42 and 76. The neuropsychological deterioration seemed to persist until the age of four to five years, plateauing later without further regression. All patients required early intervention and special education.

• *Caraballo and Fejerman (2006)* reported 53 patients followed until a mean age of 11 years. Mental delay was mild in 18 childhren (34%), moderate in 21 (40%), and severe in 14 (26%). Expressive and receptive dysphasia was observed in eight patients, hyperactivity in 45, and autism in two. However, the age range was large (4-14 years) and the ages at evaluation were not detailed.

• A patient with normal cognitive outcome was reported by *Buoni et al. (2006)*; a 13-year-old boy with SMEI, with two previous episodes of status epilepticus and a *de novo* truncation mutation of the *SCN1A* gene. At age 13 years, he had an IQ of 125 (WISC-R). The authors attributed this unusual good outcome to the progressive seizure reduction after the age of four.

Recent Neuropsychological Studies

• *A neuropsychological study was conducted in Marseille* (Cassé-Perrot *et al.*, 2001; Wolff *et al.*, 2006) on 20 patients aged from 11 months to 16 years and seven months, with a follow-up of over three years in 10 cases. Cognitive and behavioural difficulties were always present, but at varying degrees *(Figure 19)*.

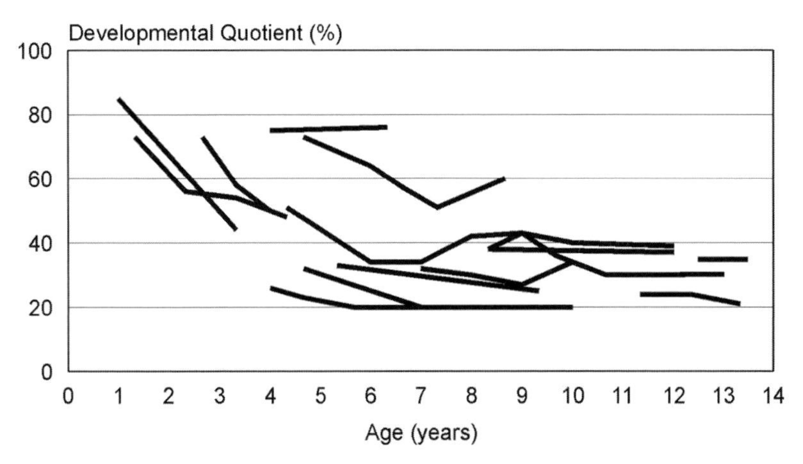

Figure 19. *Evolution of developmental quotient (from Wolff* et al., *2006).*

Neuropsychological deficits concerned all skills; motor, linguistic and visual abilities being strikingly affected. In the visuo-construction domain, the global mode of organising visual information was more affected than the piecemeal approach to construction. Behaviour was marked by hyperactivity and a psychotic nature of relationships and, sometimes, autistic traits. The appearance of neuropsychological disorders seemed to be related to the severity of the epilepsy during the first two years of life. Children with an initial high frequency of convulsive seizures showed earlier slowing of psychomotor development compared to those with fewer seizures in the first two years. There was also some relationship between the total number of convulsive seizures, their duration and the degree of mental deterioration. Three children had a better development and their language was more preserved, even if their progress exhibited a disharmonic mode. This correlated with milder epilepsy, or a marked decrease in the number of convulsive seizures from the age of six years. One child had an increasing number of seizures after the age of six years without cognitive slowing or change in behaviour. This might be explained by a greater impact of seizures on development in the first years of life. Thus, stagnation or deterioration was the rule during the first six years, but a positive evolution, albeit disharmonic, was observed thereafter and some patients could attend specialised schools or sheltered work institutions.

• *Riva et al. (2009)* studied two patients, followed from 11 months and 23 months, until seven years and six months, and eight years and six months, respectively, with repeat assessment using the Griffiths Mental Development Scales. In spite of a different epilepsy history and a less severe epilepsy course for the second patient, there appeared to be a similar progressive decline of DQ for both patients, with scores below 50 in all six domains, at the last assessment. Although the authors provided a good chronology of the history for these patients, the onset age of epilepsy and the interval between the onset and the first assessment were not indicated. Thus, it is difficult to understand the extent of developmental delay the patients already had in the first year. The authors did not consider possible differences in treatment and did not closely correlate clinical events and neuropsychological findings. However, as both patients carried a truncation mutation in the *SCN1A* gene, the authors emphasised the role of the mutation *per se* in the cognitive impairment observed in DS.

• *Ragona et al. (2010)* reported an interesting study of 37 patients referred for developmental and cognitive assessments. They divided their patients into three groups, according to the age at testing. Analysis of the results showed that the percentage of patients with severe mental retardation increased with increasing age *(Figure 20)*. In group 1 (16 patients evaluated at older than 10 years), 10 patients could not collaborate because of a very low cognitive level or behavioural disorders, two had severe retardation and only four had mild or moderate retardation. In contrast, in group 2 (six patients evaluated between seven and 10 years of age), cognitive delay was severe only in one patient, moderate in two and mild in three. In group 3 (15 patients who had their last evaluation at a younger age; between six months and six years), developmental delay became evident from the second year of life with heterogeneous levels; from severe delay (two cases) to moderate (three cases), mild (five cases) and even normal between five and six years (two cases), the remaining three were younger than three years.

The authors commented that there was no true deterioration during childhood. Indeed, developmental skills slowed down or stagnated before the age of five and remained rather stable thereafter. The decline in IQ was related to the growing gap between increasing age and steady mental ages, and by the increasing motor and behavioural disorders.

• *Ragona et al. (2011)* performed a *retrospective, multicentre study* in order to confirm the previous data and determine the factors causing the cognitive deficits observed in most patients with DS. The series included 26 patients from six different centres, observed at the onset of seizures and followed until at least the age of four. Serial awake and sleep EEGs, with polygraphy and video recording, MRI, and molecular analysis for *SCN1A,* were obtained in all cases. Serial standardised evaluations included the Griffiths or Brunet-Lézine Scales and WIPSSI, according to age and applicability. Seizure types, mean frequency and frequency variance were reviewed with attention to occurrence of status and myoclonic seizures. The effects of epilepsy and genetic variables on cognitive level were assessed by various General

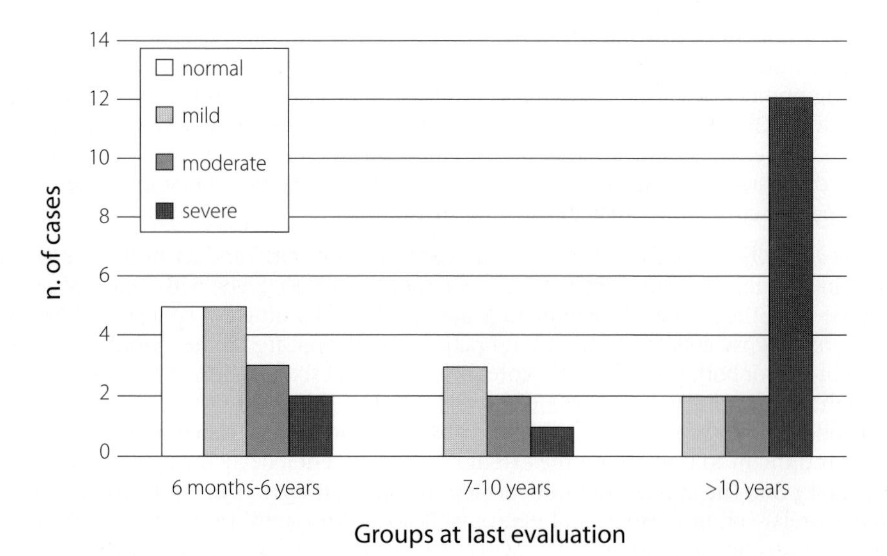

Figure 20. *Global quotient and age (from Ragona* et al., *2010). With permission.*

Linear Models (GLM). A progressive deterioration of cognitive performance with increasing age was observed in twenty patients, whereas in seven, cognitive skills remained within the low average limits at the age of four *(Figure 21).*

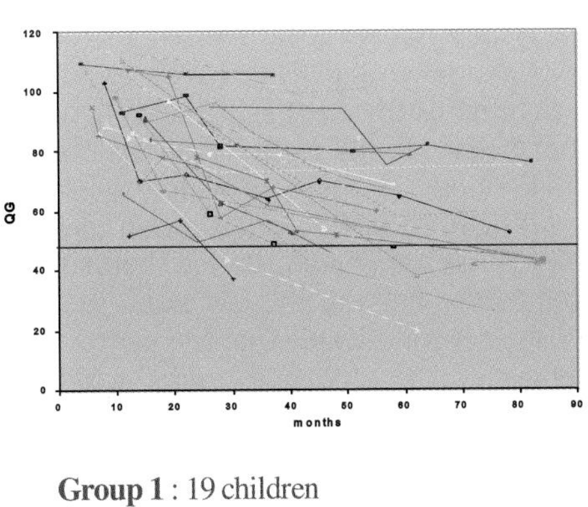

Group 1 : 19 children
onset 5,3 ± months

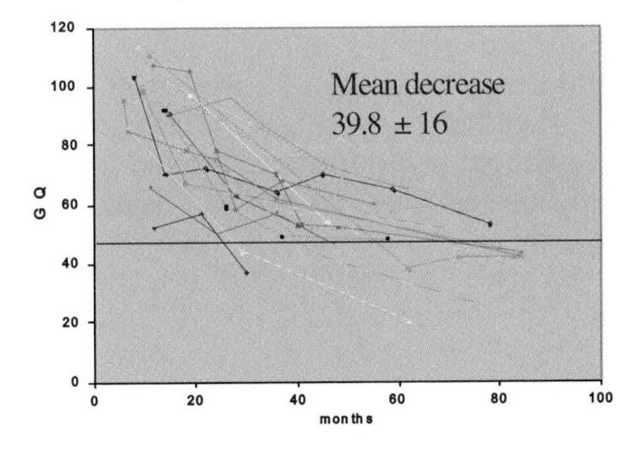

Group 2 : 7 children
onset 6,5 ± months

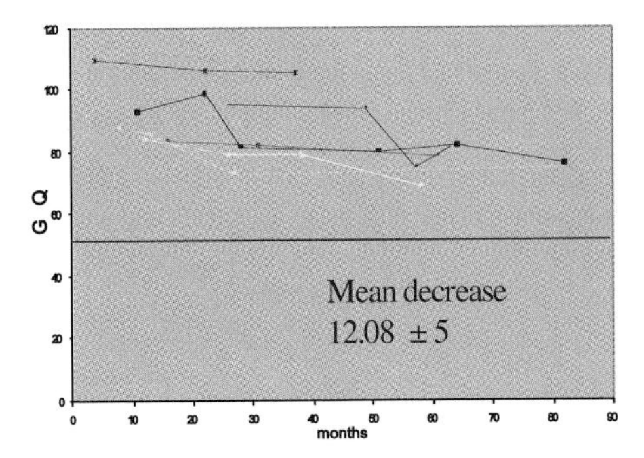

Figure 21. *GQ and age in all and in two sub-groups (from Ragona* et al., *2011).*
In Groupe 2, with a minor decline, only 1/7 patients presented with myoclonic seizures and atypical absences, apposed to 12/19 in Group 1.

On the whole, these data suggest that the epileptic phenotype contributes in determining cognitive development, and that the early appearance of myoclonus and/or absences might have a negative prognostic impact. However, the wide range of cognitive decline suggests that, beside seizures, other variables, including antiepileptic drug treatment, rehabilitation, and familial environment, greatly impact cognitive skills. Moreover, the variability of outcome and the appearance of neurological deficits, hardly ascribable to epileptic activity (*e.g.* ataxia), suggest that the channelopathy itself is probably crucial in determining the phenotype. The role of channelopathies in inducing symptoms other than seizures is well documented in the mouse genetic model of SMEI, in which the selective failure of excitability of GABAergic neurons, resulting from *SCN1A* mutations, underlies both epilepsy and motor deficits (Kalume *et al.*, 2007). It has been demonstrated that reduced excitability of cerebellar Purkinje neurons, observed in the mutant mice, is alone sufficient to cause ataxia (Grusser-Cornehls & Baurle, 2001). It is conceivable that the genetic determinants (type of mutations, modulating and epigenetic factors) may underlie different epilepsy and mental phenotypes, and that epilepsy is only one of the variables which concur in determining the final outcome.

- *Chieffo et al. (2011a)* performed an original study to assess the onset of neurodevelopmental abnormalities, including abnormalities of visual function and behaviour, in a small cohort of five children with DS. Four were selected among a cohort of infants with severe febrile seizures and followed longitudinally for possible emergence of DS, while the remaining case was studied at a later stage when there were already clear signs of the syndrome. Three of them had a borderline form without myoclonic seizures. Age at follow-up varied from 30 to 51 months. Neurodevelopmental outcome was assessed using the Griffiths Mental Scales. Visual function assessment included the following items: ocular motility, attention over distance, acuity, binocular visual fields, the fixation shift test, and stereopsis. After 18 months, behavioural problems were scored using the Achenbach Child Behavior Checklist for ages one and a half to five (CBCL/1‰-5). In these patients, cognitive deterioration appeared slightly later than previously reported; at 24, 32, 39, and 51 months, whereas in one case the DQ values were still optimal at 51 months. More interesting is the detailed assessment of various aspects of visual function. This showed that four children, when assessed in the second year or in the first half of the third year, had a diffuse involvement of most, if not all, of the explored aspects of visual function. In these cases, the abnormalities of visual function preceded those of the neurodevelopmental scale, to some extent heralding the beginning of neurocognitive involvement. An atypical course was observed in the fifth case which never showed cognitive decline or visual impairment, even at 51 months.

Four out of the five cases did not carry mutation in the *SCN1A* gene, whereas in the fifth case, a truncation mutation was found. Even though truncation mutations are often associated with a severe phenotype, in this patient DQ was within the normal range until age 30 months, in the absence of behaviour disorders, and declined only between 30 and 51 months.

The predictive value of impaired visual function versus cognitive development has been previously shown in early brain-injured infants (Mercuri *et al.*, 1999) or infants with West syndrome (Guzzetta *et al.*, 2008). The later onset of visual impairment in DS, when cognitive development is already established, could account for a developmental delay that rarely shapes the early and catastrophic profile of West syndrome.

The preliminary data suggest that early and sequential assessments of visual function should be performed as early as possible in these patients and that there is a degree of variability of neurodevelopmental outcome that should be explored further. The presence of an impairment of visual function preceding the cognitive decline could provide useful prognostic information, as well as some clues for a better understanding of the mechanisms of cognitive deterioration in this syndrome.

• *Another study by the same authors (Chieffo et al., 2011b)*, comprising 12 children, confirms that neurodevelopment in the first years of the disease is heterogeneous and does not always lead to a severe deficit. Five patients were followed beyond the age of four, up to nine years. All DQ values were below the normal range, but none in the severe mental retardation range *(Figure 22)*. One girl had reached a borderline IQ level at the age of eight and was able to learn writing, reading and counting. In all patients, impairment was more evident in hand-eye coordination, visual attention, expressive language, memory and executive functions. Longitudinal observation revealed partial recovery of language functions, and, to a lesser degree, visual attention in all cases. Conversely, mild improvement in visual motor integration was observed only in two cases. Distractibility, hyperactivity and oppositivity were observed in all patients at the first evaluation, but improved later.

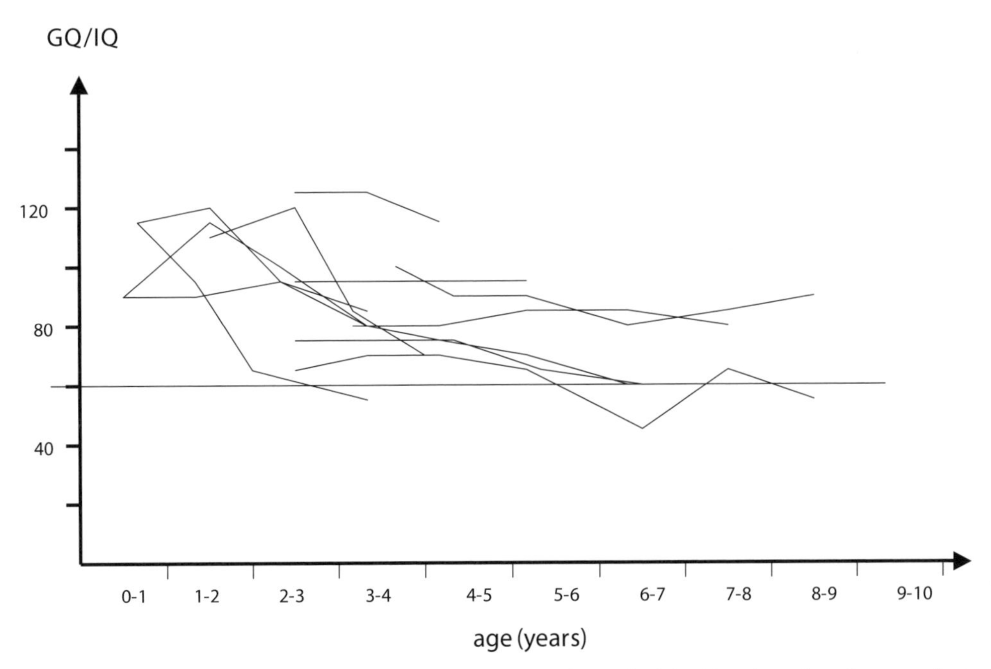

Figure 22. *Evolution of GQ (Griffiths scale) and IQ (WIPSI and WISC) of the 12 patients. In only two patients GQ or IQ declines below the level of 60 (from Chieffo* et al., *2011b).*

To summarise, all authors confirm an apparently normal early development and subsequent decline, associated with behavioural disturbances, which begins several months after the onset of seizures and ends in cognitive impairment of variable degree during childhood. In earlier reports, this decline was usually severe, whereas in recent series it was reported to be heterogeneous and patients had sometimes only mild or moderate deficits. Accurate neuropsychological studies show that some specific functions, such as visuo-perception, hand-eye coordination, expressive language, and executive functions are more impaired than other functions. Attention deficit is the most constant and precocious trait. Hyperactivity is also observed during the second year of life. Clumsiness becomes obvious later on. Many children present with relational difficulties, sometimes of a psychotic type. Although autistic traits are often observed, only a few children are actually autistic.

4. Neuroimaging and neuropathology

A main question in Dravet syndrome is whether the behavioural problems and cognitive impairment that emerge after the brain has experienced early prolonged febrile convulsive and non-convulsive seizures, often manifested as multiple intractable seizure types, is related to seizure induced brain damage (Guerrini & Falchi, 2011). Examples have been reported of families in which amongst multiple individuals carrying *SCN1A* gene mutations, those having experienced a limited number of seizures have normal cognition while those with intractable seizures are cognitively impaired (Suls *et al.*, 2010; Guerrini *et al.*, 2010). Ataxic gait, or motor awkwardness and hyperactivity, and a jerky movement pattern are also reported in many of the children who have suffered severe seizures. It has become obvious that the underlying genetic defect confers a peculiar profile of seizure susceptibility but is not the sole determinant of severity. Since the genetic abnormality does not appear sufficient to cause the impairment *per se*, it is plausible to hypothesize that other factors, possibly seizure related structural changes might contribute to producing cognitive impairment.

EEGs may be normal at onset but background activity can later deteriorate and generalized and multifocal abnormalities, such as spikes, spike-waves, polyspikes and slow waves, appear. It has been suggested that preserved background activity correlates with milder cognitive impairment (Akiyama *et al.*, 2010). There are only a few available data on morphologic or functional neuroimaging as well as neuropathology in Dravet syndrome and is therefore difficult to argue to what extent differences in cognitive and motor impairment have a structural anatomic counterpart.

MRI findings

No gross abnormalities were detected on early brain CT or MRI studies, although signs of slight or moderate, diffuse, cerebral or cerebellar atrophy, increased white matter signal, were occasionally reported (Dalla Bernardina *et al.*, 1982; Dravet *et al.*, 2005a, b). In a few patients, neuroimaging was normal at the onset but brain atrophy appeared during follow-up (Dravet *et al.*, 2005a, b). Only two studies, both retrospective, have systematically investigated MRI findings (Siegler *et al.*, 2005; Striano *et al.*, 2007a). Siegler *et al.* (2005) studied a series of patients in whom no mutation analysis of the *SCN1A* gene had been performed. These authors found MRI changes consistent with hippocampal sclerosis (HS) in 10 out of 14 children with a clinical diagnosis of DS, aged 1.2 to 16 years (mean: 7.2). In six, who had been reported to have normal earlier MRI scans, HS had become obvious on a repeat scan. None of the

10 patients exhibited the clinical features of mesial temporal lobe epilepsy. Cerebral or cerebellar atrophy were observed in six out of 14 adult patients; one also exhibiting imaging evidence of hippocampal sclerosis (Jansen *et al.*, 2006).

Striano and colleagues (2007a) reviewed the MRI data of 58 patients (35 with a *SCN1A* mutation) in whom the last scan had been performed at 1.5-T after the age of four years. A detailed study of the hippocampal regions was available in all. Thirteen patients (22.4%) had MRI findings that were considered as abnormal; three patients had enlarged ventricles; one had unilateral HS and one had focal cortical dysplasia *(Figure 23)*. Duration of epilepsy and age at seizure onset did not correlate with the presence of MRI abnormalities. There was no correlation between abnormal MRIs and the frequency of episodes of status epilepticus having occurred within the first four years of life. Abnormal findings were more frequently observed in patients without *SCN1A* mutations (39.1% *vs.* 11.4%; $p = 0.02$). Absence of mutations in a specific gene makes the latter subgroup likely to be etiologically heterogeneous, however.

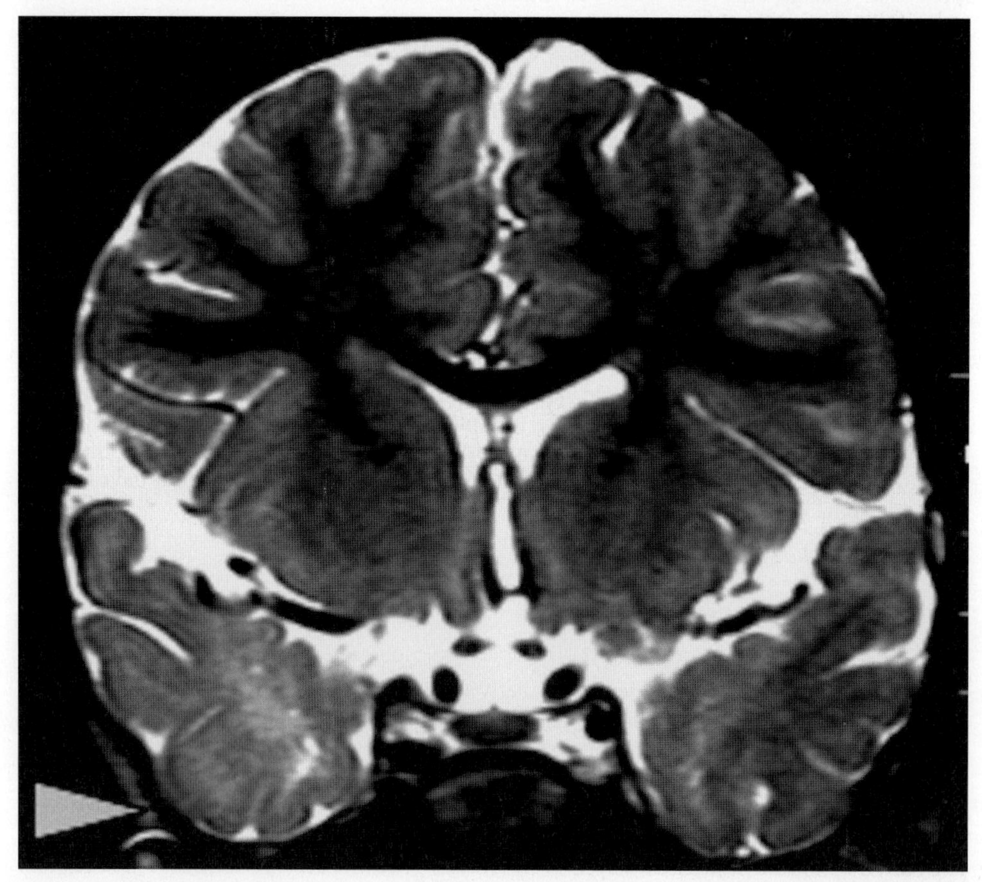

Figure 23. *High signal intensity abnormality of the right temporal pole in a three year old boy with a SCN1A mutation and repeated episodes of left unilateral clonic status epilepticus triggered by fever and of complex partial seizures of right temporal lobe origin. This image is consistent with focal cortical dysplasia. Coronal T_2-weighted image.*

SPECT findings

Only a few SPECT or PET studies have been performed in Dravet syndrome. A SPECT study (Nieto-Barrera *et al.*, 2000a) showed areas of hypoperfusion in eight out of 10 patients; the finding was limited to one hemisphere in five patients and was bilateral in the remaining three. Areas of hypoperfusion did not clearly correlate with EEG findings.

Neuropathology

The first available neuropathologic study that was said to have been performed in Dravet syndrome was carried on a 19-month-old boy who had died unexpectedly (Renier & Renkawek, 1990). The most striking features included microdysgenesis of the cerebellum and the cerebral cortex and threefold spinal cord channels with surrounding ectopic tissue. The hippocampus and brainstem were normal. An additional autopsy case was reported in a 7-year-old girl who had died of haemorrhagic shock precipitated by an influenza infection (Hayashi *et al.*, 2004). Reported findings included oedema and ischemic changes, related to the haemorrhagic shock, as well as fused gyri and heterotopic neurons in the adjacent white matter in the frontal and parietal cortex. The hippocampus harboured mild gliosis in the endplate (CA4), and calcified foci were present in the globus pallidus. Myelinated fibers were reduced in the spinal pyramidal tracts.

The origin of these subtle structural changes, which in neither of the two patients were visible by imaging, remains unclear. Furthermore, it is not known whether a *SCN1A* mutation was present in these two patients.

Le Gal *et al.* (2010) found multifocal micronodular dysplasia of the left temporal cortex and bilateral endfolium gliosis on a neuropathological study of the whole brain of a child with Dravet syndrome and a *SCN1A* abnormality. In an extensive post mortem neuropathological study of three adult cases, no histological signature of the condition was identified; there was no evidence of cerebral neurodegeneration (Catarino *et al.*, unpublished observations, quoted in Guerrini *et al.*, 2011).

The uncertain meaning of structural changes

Neuroimaging studies are mostly unrevealing and neuropathological studies are extremely limited in Dravet syndrome. Correctness of diagnosis is doubtful in the cases included in some earlier studies in which no genetic testing was performed, leaving uncertainty about the reported findings.

The study by Striano *et al.* (2007a) provided reliable information on a relatively well characterized population, demonstrating that abnormal MRI findings only occur in a small minority of patients, confirming that epilepsy in Dravet syndrome has a functional rather than structural basis. On the other hand, the origin of structural abnormalities, such focal brain atrophy, cortical dysplasia, and HS, in some children with *SCN1A* mutations remains unclear. Putative underlying mechanisms for brain atrophy include Wallerian degeneration, apoptotic cell death, inflammation, and excitotoxicity, whereas prolonged febrile seizures might be responsible for HS (Guerrini *et al.*, 2011). While in some patients, no focal neurological manifestations, focal seizures or EEG abnormalities are observed in keeping with the site of the MRI abnormalities, which are therefore likely incidental, in other patients the expression of epilepsy appears to be influenced by a focal structural abnormality, with most seizures and EEG abnormalities originating from the site of the structural change (Guerrini *et al.*, 2011) *(Figures 24 and 25)*. Prospective quantitative neuroimaging studies, including volumetric evaluations, might be able to assess the etiological role of the changes observed in these patients. Chipaux and colleagues (2010) reported unusual anoxoischemic-like MRI lesions in three patients with *SCN1A* mutations and Dravet syndrome who following refractory status epilepticus had experienced persistent, severe cognitive and motor deterioration. These MRI abnormalities could not be explained by hemodynamic failure but no plausible causative mechanism could be identified.

Sakakibara *et al.* (2009) reported a two-year-old girl who had experienced repeated episodes of febrile status epilepticus during infancy and myoclonus, consistent with a clinical diagnosis of Dravet syndrome and a nonsense mutation in *SCN1A*, developing persistent right hemiclonic seizures and left unilateral cortical laminar necrosis followed by progressive cerebral atrophy at age 15 months. The clinical and neuroradiological picture was consistent with the

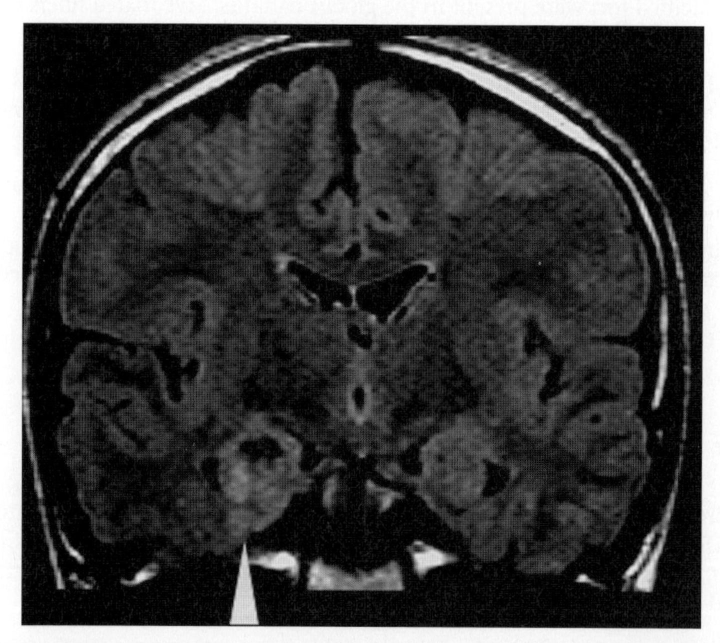

Figure 24. *Coronal FLAIR image. 16 year old boy with a truncating mutation of the SCN1A gene [p. Arg580X (R580X)] and right hippocampal sclerosis (arrow). First febrile seizure at 10 months. Then one to four seizures/ year, without fever: Right version, left sided jerks and vomiting. QIV: 78; QIP: 54; QIT: 64. This clinical picture is indicative of focal epilepsy with fever sensitivity and seizure origin in the right hemisphere.*

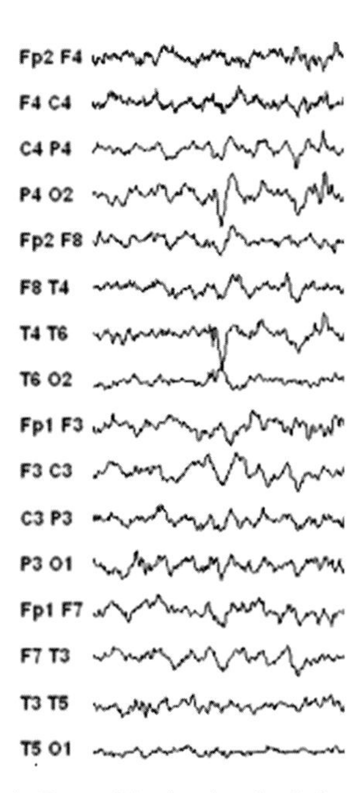

Figure 25. *EEG of the same patient as in* Figure 23, *showing focal abnormalities in the right temporo-occipital leads.*

hemiconvulsion-hemiplegia (HH) syndrome. This observation confirms the potential, though exceedingly rare, risk in children with Dravet syndrome to develop structural changes that can, in turn, be the substrate for the epileptic encephalopathy.

Ohmori *et al.* (2008) reported a patient with typical Rasmussen encephalitis in whom a *SCN1A*-R1575C mutation (carried by the unaffected father) was fortuitously identified. The R1575C mutant channels transiently expressed in human embryonic kidney exhibited defective electrophysiological properties. Although it is possible that this association be coincidental, this observation opens interesting perspectives about the genetic-environment interaction in relation to an autoimmune-mediated brain disorder. Furthermore, the underlying dysfunction of the *SCN1A* gene might confer to the brain a unique profile of vulnerability whose consequences are not easily disclosed by neuropathology. For example it has been demonstrated that seizure induced changes may affect selective cell subpopulations and require specific experimental settings to be fully appreciated in their extent and consequences (Liu *et al.*, 2003). Prospective studies will clarify to what extent earlier diagnosis and efforts at seizure control with more appropriate drug combinations may influence the development of clinical deterioration. Animal models may, in turn, help clarifying the role of pathological deterioration, if any, and of its prevention by improved seizure control.

5. The genetics of Dravet syndrome

In collaboration with Carla Marini

Paediatric Neurology Unit and Laboratories, Children's Hospital A. Meyer, University of Florence, Firenze, Italy

Sodium channel α1 and Dravet Syndrome

A clinical diagnosis of Dravet syndrome is supported by the finding of the α1 subunit of the sodium channel (*SCN1A)* gene mutations in most patients. Voltage gated sodium channels (VGSCs) are required for the initiation and propagation of action potentials. Mutations of the *SCN1A* gene were first discovered in the epilepsy syndrome of genetic (formerly generalized) epilepsy with febrile seizure plus (GEFS+) (Escayg *et al.*, 2000). A family history of epilepsy or febrile seizures is sometimes found in patients with Dravet syndrome and most affected relatives have GEFS+ phenotypes (Singh *et al.*, 2001). In view of the predisposition to seizures with fever that typically occurs in Dravet syndrome, Claes and colleagues performed mutation analysis on *SCN1A* in seven children, all of whom turned out to harbour *de novo* mutations (Claes *et al.*, 2001).

More than 700 mutations have then been associated with Dravet syndrome. These mutations are randomly distributed across the SCN1A protein, as they are in (GEFS+) (Mulley *et al.*, 2006; Marini *et al.*, 2007; Depienne *et al.*, 2009a). The frequency of *SCN1A* alterations in Dravet syndrome is around 85%. By classical Sanger sequencing, mutations are found in about 80% of cases and comprise truncating (40%) and missense mutations (40%) with the remaining being splice site changes. Most mutations are *de novo*, but familial mutations occur in 5-10% of cases and are usually missense in nature (Claes *et al.*, 2001; Nabbout *et al.*, 2003; Wallace *et al.*, 2003; Fujiwara *et al.*, 2003). In these cases, the proband, through which the family was ascertained, usually has a severe phenotype, while the remaining family members with the same mutation have milder phenotypes, consistent with the GEFS+ spectrum (Nabbout *et al.*, 2003; Fujiwara *et al.*, 2003). Several families have been reported with more than one child with Dravet syndrome. This occurrence has important genetic counselling consequences as the syndrome can be transmitted from an unaffected, or mildly affected parent, to one or more severely affected children through somatic or germline mosaic mutations in the transmitting parent (Depienne *et al.*, 2006; Marini *et al.*, 2006; Gennaro *et al.*, 2006; Morimoto *et al.*, 2006; Vadlamudi *et al.*, 2010). This mechanism seems to be at play in at least 7% of families with Dravet syndrome (Depienne *et al.*, 2010). The proportion of the mutated allele in the blood of the Dravet syndrome patients described varied from 0.04-85% and may be a significant factor underlying intra-familial phenotypic variability (Depienne *et al.*, 2010). De novo mutations occur indeed at any time, from the premorula stage of the embryo, causing disease and the highest proportion of mutated allele, to adulthood, with mutations in germ-line cells of healthy parents, causing disease in the offspring (Vadlamudi *et al.*, 2010).

Patients with a clinical diagnosis of DS who test negative for *SCN1A* mutations after sequencing may still have exonic deletions or chromosomal rearrangements involving *SCN1A* (Mulley *et al.*, 2006; Marini *et al.*, 2007; Suls *et al.*, 2006; Madia *et al.*, 2006; Wang *et al.*, 2008). The size of these genomic alterations varies from the megabase range, involving a large number of contiguous genes, down to one exon within *SCN1A (Figure 26)*. Duplications and amplifications involving *SCN1A* are additional, rare, molecular mechanisms (Marini *et al.*, 2009). Such abnormalities can be identified with multiplex ligation-dependent probe amplification (MPLA) and further characterized by comparative genome hybridization (CGH) to determine the size of the abnormality and identify any additional gene(s) involved (Marini *et al.*, 2009). Haplotype analysis with microsatellite markers and single nucleotide polymorphisms (SNPs) and multiplex amplicon quantification (MAQ) can also be used to identify small chromosomal abnormalities affecting *SCN1A* (Madia *et al.*, 2006; Suls *et al.*, 2006). Intragenic and whole gene deletions including *SCN1A* and/or contiguous genes account for 2-3% of Dravet syndrome cases and for about 12.5% of those who are mutation-negative on classical Sanger sequencing (Marini *et al.*, 2009). It has been suggested that microchromosomal rearrangements extending beyond *SCN1A* and including a variable number of contiguous genes may be potentially associated with additional dysmorphic features (Madia *et al.*, 2006), depending on the genes involved, or, possibly, with a more severe epilepsy phenotype when other ***VGSC*** α subunit genes clustered on chromosome 2q such as *SCN2A, SCN3A, SCN7A* and *SCN9A* are involved (Pereira *et al.*, 2004; Davidsson *et al.*, 2008). However, attempts at defining genotype – phenotype correlations based on the size of the underlying deletions have provided inconsistent findings. Pereira *et al.* (2004) suggested the epilepsy phenotype to be particularly severe and dysmorphic features to be an additional phenotypic trait in one patient with a large chromosome 2q deletion involving both *SCN1A* and *SCN2A*. Suls *et al.* (2006) described three patients with microchromosomal rearrangements extending beyond *SCN1A*; while two of them exhibited additional clinical features, the third did not, suggesting that haploinsufficiency of the additionally deleted genes did not result in overt features in that patient (Suls *et al.*, 2006). Other studies have shown that no remarkable clinical differences can be appreciated between patients with Dravet syndrome in whom a deletion only involves *SCN1A* and those in whom contiguous genes were also removed (Mulley *et al.*, 2006, Marini *et al.*, 2009). So, although haploinsufficiency of more than voltage gated sodium channel α, subunit gene might be expected to cause a more severe epilepsy phenotype, patients with large deletions including additional subunit genes most often exhibit a phenotype similar to those carrying point mutations (Marini *et al.*, 2009). It is also possible that clinical differences that may be due to nearby genes become negligeable within the severe clinical context of Dravet syndrome.

Nakayama *et al.* (2010) reported two patients harbouring heterozygous microdeletions removing the 5′ noncoding exons and regions with promoter activity but not affecting the coding exons. These findings further confirm the critical and predominant involvement of *SCN1A* in the molecular pathology of the syndrome.

In families where the proband with Dravet syndrome has a *de novo SCN1A* mutation but other relatives have epilepsy or febrile seizures, the mode of inheritance is likely to be polygenic and *SCN1A* is one of the genetic determinants specifically associated with Dravet syndrome but not with the other phenotypes. A patient with Dravet syndrome with genetic variants in both *SCN1A* and *SCN9A* has been reported, suggesting that mutations of *SCN9A*

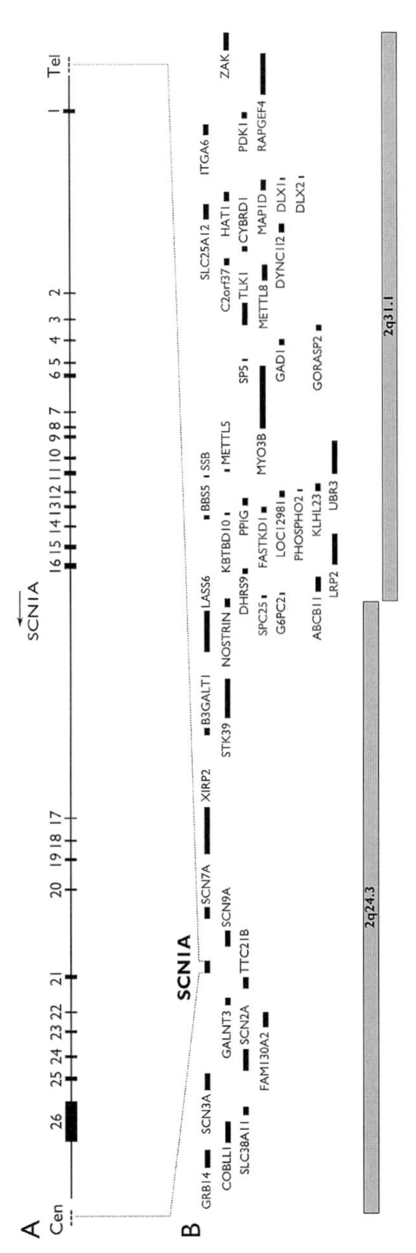

Figure 26. *Microchromosomal abnormalities characterized by multiplex ligation-dependent probe amplification (MLPA) and array comparative gene hybridization (CGH).* ***(A)*** *Magnification of SCN1A intragenic single or multiple exon deletions identified by MLPA in the series reported by Marini* et al. *(2009).* ***(B)*** *Gene content of deletions extending beyond SCN1A and spanning with a variable extent from 2q24.3 to 2q31.1, as further characterized by array CGH. (From Marini* et al.*, 2009, modified).*

might cause FS and be modifiers for the Dravet syndrome phenotype; a finding that needs to be confirmed but which might provide support for the role of additional genes modifying a gene of major effect (*SCN1A*) (Singh *et al.*, 2009).

Dravet syndrome without *SCN1A* alterations

Mutations of protocadherin 19 (*PCDH19*, on chromosome Xq22) have been associated with "epilepsy and mental retardation limited to females" (EFMR) (OMIM#300088) (Scheffer *et al.*, 2008; Dibbens *et al.*, 2008). EFMR exhibits an unusual X-linked inheritance pattern, where the disorder is expressed in heterozygous females whereas hemizygous males are unaffected carriers (Dibbens *et al.*, 2008). *PCDH19* is expressed in developing brains of humans and mice, and is postulated to be involved in establishing neuronal connections and signal transduction at the synaptic membrane level (Yagi *et al.*, 2000) and molecular specification of neurons in the cerebral cortex (Krishna *et al.*, 2011).

Depienne *et al.* reported *PCDH19* familial and "de novo„ point mutations in 13 females with early onset epileptic encephalopathy mimicking Dravet syndrome (Depienne *et al.*, 2009b). The study was prompted by the observation of a boy with a similar phenotype who carried a mosaic chromosomal rearrangement leading to *PCDH19* haploinsufficiency. The authors estimated that 16%, or 25% if only females were included, of their *SCN1A* mutation-negative Dravet syndrome patients had *PCDH19* mutations and that this gene might overall account for 5% of DS (Depienne *et al.*, 2009b). In a subsequent study, mutation screening of a large cohort of females with variable epilepsy phenotypes with infantile onset, revealed *PCDH19* mutations in 13 probands, seven of whom were reported to exhibit a Dravet syndrome phenotype and six having focal epilepsy (Marini *et al.*, 2010). Clinical features observed in some of the patients with *PCDH19* mutations and in those with Dravet syndrome due to *SCN1A* mutations, including infantile onset of febrile and afebrile seizures, seizures in clusters during fever, regression following seizure onset, suggest that *PCDH19* should be tested in Dravet syndrome patients who are negative on screening for mutations or genomic abnormalities of *SCN1A*. However, the electroclinical features observed in girls with *PCDH19* mutations have not been reported in detail and no clear pattern is known to occur that can be compared to those known to occur in Dravet syndrome. It is possible that as descriptions of EEG characteristics and video-EEG recorded seizure patterns in *PCDH19* mutated girls will become available, differences will emerge that are now not recognizable based on clinical descriptions alone.

A single case of DS with a mutation in the α2 subunit gene of the $GABA_A$ receptor, *GABRG2*, has been reported (Harkin *et al.*, 2002). Patino and co-authors (2009) reported a single patient with DS carrying a homozygous mutation in *SCN1B*. This is the only Dravet syndrome patient with an autosomal recessive pattern of inheritance.

Genotype-phenotype correlations

SCN1A mutations have been predominantly associated with Dravet syndrome and the GEFS+ spectrum and are characterised by phenotypic variability, including age of seizure onset, seizure types and severity, as well as variable cognitive outcome. Although mutations, or deletions, in the same gene may result in different phenotypes, some general genotype-phenotype correlations have been attempted. Truncating, nonsense, frame shift mutations and partial or whole gene deletions usually cause a classical Dravet syndrome phenotype and appear to be correlated with an earlier age at seizure onset (Marini *et al.*, 2007). However, in Dravet syndrome, *SCN1A* truncation mutations account for 40% of mutations and missense mutations account for another 40% (Depienne *et al.*, 2009a). The severity of the phenotypes is also correlated with the location of *SCN1A* missense mutations: for example, those in the pore-forming region of the sodium channel may cause Dravet syndrome *(Figure 27)*, while those missense changes located outside the pore-forming region are rather associated with the GEFS+ spectrum (Meisler & Kearney, 2005). However, a genotype-phenotype correlation is not consistently observed as, for example, the same *SCN1A* mutations and deletions cause Dravet syndrome in some patients and GEFS+ in others (Escayg *et al.*, 2000; Suls *et al.*, 2010; Guerrini *et al.*, 2010). Even in the presence of a genomic deletion, whose effects are comparable to those of a truncation mutation and would be expected to result in a uniformly severe clinical picture, the associated phenotype may vary so that individuals with mild epilepsy and no cognitive impairment can be observed next to individuals with severe cognitive impairment and Dravet syndrome, even within the same family (Suls *et al.*, 2010; Guerrini *et al.*, 2010). Remarkable variability in phenotype severity within a single family favours the concept that *SCN1A* loss of function causes a spectrum of epilepsy and cognitive phenotypes in which seizures precipitated by fever are the prominent feature and schematic subdivisions would be inappropriate. These observations also strongly suggest that modifier genes, the genetic background and/or environmental factors may play a role in some patients, and thus Dravet syndrome may sometimes follow a complex model of inheritance. Overall, studies addressing correlations between *SCN1A* gene alterations and phenotype severity in large series have failed to find a reliable correspondence (Wallace *et al.*, 2003; Fukuma *et al.*, 2004; Oguni *et al.*, 2005).

SCN1A MUTATIONS ASSOCIATED WITH OTHER FORMS OF EPILEPSY AND WITH NON-EPILEPSY PHENOTYPES

"Borderline severe myoclonic epilepsy of infancy" (SMEB) refers to patients who lack some of the "key" features of DS, such as myoclonic seizures or generalized spike and wave activity. More than 70% of SMEB patients carry *SCN1A* mutations, which are spread throughout the gene with a mixture of mutations including truncating, missense and splice site changes (Harkin *et al.*, 2007).

Infants with frequent and intractable generalized tonic-clonic seizures (ICEGTC) (Fujiwara *et al.*, 2003) follow a similar developmental course as children with Dravet syndrome, including developmental slowing in the second year of life and poor cognitive outcome. The major feature that differentiates Dravet syndrome and ICEGTC is the presence of other seizure types such as myoclonic, absence and complex partial seizures. These patients also have a high frequency of *SCN1A* mutations (Fujiwara *et al.*, 2003).

Five patients with early onset multifocal seizures, developmental slowing and abundant multifocal epileptiform activity have been designated as "severe infantile multifocal

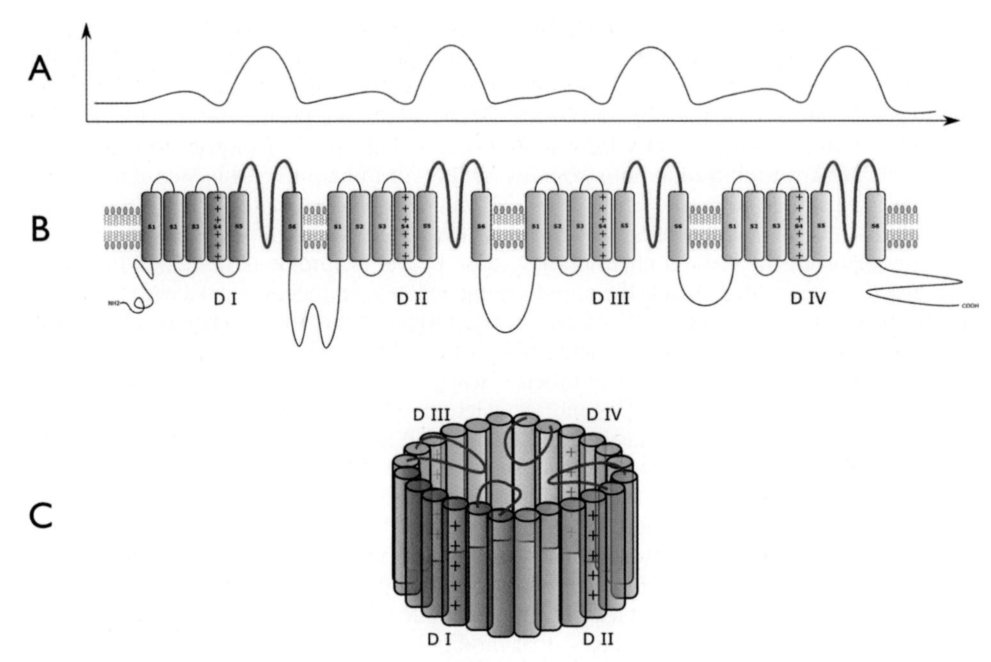

Figure 27. ***(B)** Graphic representation of the SCN1A protein showing the four transmembrane domains (D I – D IV) and pore forming regions. Mutations leading to truncated SCN1A protein and to mRNA splicing alteration, associated with Dravet syndrome, can occur at any site. A tridimentional representation of the SCN1A channel is shown in C. In the upper part of the figure **(A)**, a graphic provides a quantitative representation of the location of missense mutations causing Dravet syndrome with respect to the domains where they occur, as represented just below in **B**. It is immediately evident that most Dravet syndrome causing missense mutations fall within the pore forming regions of the protein.*

epilepsy" (SIMFE); the three with normal early development carried *SCN1A* mutations while the two with developmental delay predating seizures did not (Harkin *et al.*, 2007). The clinical keys that distinguish these patients from Dravet syndrome, would be a focal form of epilepsy, rather than generalized, rare myoclonic and absence seizures and the lack of GSW on EEG.

The identification of *SCN1A* mutations in similar proportions of classical Dravet syndrome, SMEB, ICEGTC and SIMFE patients (Fujiwara *et al.*, 2003; Harkin *et al.*, 2007) confirms that these phenotypes share the same genetic determinant in most patients. Thus, it may be better to regard these phenotypes as a continuum of the same disorder, which could be considered the Dravet syndrome spectrum.

SCN1A missense mutations have also been associated with familial hemiplegic migraine (FHM) in a few families (Dichgans *et al.*, 2005; Vanmolkot *et al.*, 2007). Familial hemiplegic migraine is a heterogeneous disorder that has also been associated with mutations of the *CACNA1A* and *ATP1A2* genes. The missense mutation Q1489K of *SCN1A* is a recurrent mutation that results in a charge-altering aminoacid exchange in the hinged-lid domain of the protein, which is critical for fast inactivation of the channel (Dichgans *et al.*, 2005). Familial hemiplegic migraine is in turn, occasionally associated with cerebellar ataxia and epileptic seizures. Cosegregation of FHM and seizures has been associated with a missense *SCN1A* mutation (L263V) in a family in which epileptic seizures occurred independently from hemiplegic migraine attacks (Castro *et al.*, 2009). In another family the novel missense T1174S mutation was associated with "myoclonus and abnormal EEG" in a child and with hemiplegic migraine in his mother and grandmother (Gargus & Tournay, 2007).

A rare eye phenotype defined as "elicited repetitive daily blindness" (ERDB) has also been reported to be cosegregating with FHM in two families harbouring two novel missense mutations (4495T>C/p.Phe1499Leu and c.4467G>C/p.Gln1489His) located in the highly conserved intracellular loop (Vahedi *et al.*, 2009). The voltage-gated sodium channel Nav1.1 is also expressed in the retina. This peculiar eye phenotype is thought to be caused by abnormal propagation of the retinal electrical signal, which might represent retinal spreading depression.

A possible difference in the functional effect of *SCN1A* mutations leading to FHM and epilepsy has emerged from the experiments by Cestèle *et al.* (2008). These authors showed that the recurrent FHM mutation Q1489K, transfected in tsA-201 cells and cultured neurons exerted effects on the gating properties of the channel that were consistent with both hyperexcitability and hypoexcitability. Simulation of neuronal firing and long depolarizing pulses, as observed in promigraine conditions, produced effects indicating that the mutation is a gain of function, consistent with increased neuronal firing. However, during high-frequency discharges and long depolarisations, the effect became a loss of function. Recordings of firing of transfected neurons showed higher firing frequency at the beginning of long discharges. The authors hypothesized that the observed self-limited capacity to induce neuronal hyperexcitability might be a specific characteristic of migraine mutations, able to both trigger migraine and prevent the development of the extreme hyperexcitability typical of epileptic seizures.

Functional effects of voltage-gated sodium channel α1 mutations

Based on the number of patients with epilepsy in which mutations have been identified, *SCN1A* is currently considered to be the most clinically relevant epilepsy gene. The vast majority of *SCN1A* mutations responsible for GEFS+ are missense, whereas mutations responsible for Dravet syndrome can either be missense or cause truncation that would generate non-functional channels. When studied in expression systems, missense *SCN1A* mutants exhibit loss or gain of function, which are consistent with either decreased or increased neuronal excitability. However, loss of function seems to be the main effect through which *SCN1A* mutations exert their pathogenic mechanism; more than half of the identified Dravet syndrome mutants are predicted to be non-functional (Meisler & Kearney, 2005; Mulley *et al.*, 2005; Catterall *et al.*, 2008) and most missense mutations cause a reduction in Na^+ current (Ragsdale, 2008).

The fact that mutations in *SCN1A* lead to loss of function and reduced Na^+ current has initially been seen as hard to reconcile with the fact that epilepsy is an expression of brain hyperexcitability; even more so in Dravet syndrome in which hyperexcitability seems to be ubiquitous in the cortex. However, data from *Scn1a* knock-out mice (Yu *et al.*, 2006) and knock-in mice expressing the non-sense scn1a-R1407X DS mutant (Ogiwara *et al.*, 2007) have shown that the $\alpha1$ subunit is fundamental for the excitability of at least some types of GABAergic interneurons in the neocortex and hippocampus. The heterozygous Scn1a+/- mice exhibits spontaneous seizures with a remarkable dependence on the genetic background (Yu *et al.*, 2006). In this animal model, the sodium current density is substantially reduced in inhibitory GABAergic interneurons but not in the excitatory pyramidal neurons. Reduced sodium currents in inhibitory interneurons reduces their ability for sustained action potential firing, which would reduce their GABAergic output and enhance the excitability of their downstream synaptic targets, leading in turn to epilepsy. Therefore, reduced firing of inhibitory interneurons and compromised network inhibition appears to be the major pathophysiological mechanism causing *SCN1A*-related epilepsies (Martin *et al.*, 2010). The observation of variable penetration of the epileptic phenotype in different genetic backgrounds correlates with the observed variable penetrance in humans and supports the notion that modifier gene(s) are necessary for Dravet syndrome to appear. It is not known whether the primary *SCN1A* defect and modifier gene(s) might also influence cognitive functioning per se (Guerrini & Falchi, 2011).

Genetic markers and syndrome definition

When Dravet syndrome was first recognised as a clinical entity, the more severely affected patients, representing the core of the syndrome, were those attracting most of the medical attention and were therefore indentified sooner as a homogeneous group. However, recognising an underlying specific genetic defect, allows to subsequently use it to test patients whose phenotype progressively moves away from the initially defined core syndrome. The final, cumulative result of this process is the delineation of a syndrome spectrum, in which the distribution in the population of affected individuals usually corresponds to a bell shaped curve. In the middle of the curve, where most patients are represented, are the most common phenotypes, those that have led to defining the core syndrome, while at extremes are the less typical, and less frequent phenotypes (Guerrini & Oguni, 2011). Therefore, the genetic marker represented by alterations of the *SCN1A* gene has been instrumental to define the core and the ‘borderlands’ of the syndrome but has also, unavoidably, shown that a continuum exists within an entity with variable severity and often polymorphic expression, which is unpredictably influenced by additional genetic factors as well as precipitating factors. For example, in some patients, clinical manifestations are so prominently related to fever that they can experience very bad periods in which recurrent, trivial febrile illnesses precipitate severe seizures and better periods, without any febrile illness and with rare seizures. Another example, is represented by the observation that the proportion of patients with borderline SMEI who carry *SCN1A* mutations is the same as that observed in classical Dravet syndrome and that, even within a same family, the same mutation can cause both typical and ‘borderline’ forms, indicating causal homogeneity (Guerrini *et al.*, 2010; Suls *et al.*, 2010). While some authors found truncating mutations only in classical Dravet syndrome (Fukuma *et al.*, 2004), others have suggested that the types and domain distribution of mutations are similar to those observed in the borderline forms (Harkin *et al.*, 2007).

At present, when dealing with an infant who has presented more than one prolonged febrile seizure, an increasing number of clinicians would require *SCN1A* gene testing. Finding a mutation would confirm a *SCN1A* gene related disorder, leaving evolution towards either a GEFS+, or a borderline SMEI or Dravet syndrome, unpredictable, due to the lack of consistent genotype phenotype correlations. There are many reasons then why genetic diagnosis is most often of little use to predict the severity of the disorder.

6. Differential Diagnosis and Diagnostic Workup

Diagnosis

The main diagnostic criteria are: essentially a normal infant with onset in the first year of life of prolonged and repeated febrile or afebrile, generalised and unilateral clonic seizures, shortly thereafter associated with other seizure types, delayed psychomotor development and behavioural disorders, pharmacoresistance, limited (if any) abnormalities in the initial EEG, and normal brain MRI. One must keep in mind that DS is a clinical entity with a diagnosis that may be based on clinical criteria even when the genetic analysis does not reveal an abnormality of the *SCN1A* gene. Around 20% of cases do not exhibit an abnormality in the *SCN1A* gene. As the clinical symptomatology appears progressively between the first and fourth year, an early diagnosis is often difficult. In 2008, Hattori *et al.* proposed a screening test for the prediction of the syndrome before one year of age. Although this procedure is suboptimal, it is however useful and will be considered in this chapter.

Differential diagnosis

Febrile seizures. As the first clonic seizures in SMEI are often associated with fever, distinguishing them from febrile seizures is important. In SMEI, (1) onset is early, before one year of age; (2) seizures are clonic and often unilateral rather than generalised tonic-clonic or purely tonic; (3) seizures are prolonged and frequent, even when treated; and (4) body temperature is not very high. Thus, after two seizures with slight temperature elevation (from 37.5° C) and after two seizures, of which at least one is prolonged (> 5 minutes) or evolves into status, and if the infant is otherwise healthy with normal brain imaging, a diagnosis of DS should be suspected and a chronic treatment prescribed in order to prevent other prolonged seizures and status episodes. The occurrence of other convulsive seizures, with or without fever, in spite of the treatment, reinforces this suspicion. At this stage, genetic testing for *SCN1A* should be proposed. The diagnosis becomes obvious when seizures occur without fever and are associated with other seizure types (myoclonic seizures [except in SMEB], atypical absences, partial seizures, and obtundation status), or when photically-induced SWs appear, although their occurrence may be delayed for several months or years.

The findings presented by Hattori *et al.* (2008) are in keeping with our own observations. These authors compared the clinical characteristics before one year of age between two groups of infants who presented with febrile seizures within the first year: one group had been diagnosed with DS (46 patients) and the second with a different diagnosis (50 patients). Significant risk factors for DS included: age at onset of febrile seizure of seven months or less, a total number of seizures of five or more, and prolonged seizures lasting for more than 10 minutes. Other predictive factors were hemiconvulsions, partial seizures, myoclonic seizures, and hot water-induced seizures. If the total clinical risk score was ≥ 6, *SCN1A* mutation analysis was recommended *(Table II)*.

Benign myoclonic epilepsy of infancy may also begin in the first year, but is nevertheless different from DS. The main symptoms are brief myoclonic seizures appearing in a normal infant without long and repeated convulsive seizures or other seizure types. They are easily controlled by treatment. In some patients, rare simple febrile seizures can occur. Psychomotor development is normal, although some children may exhibit borderline cognitive skills at school age and slight behavioural disturbances (Dravet & Bureau, 2005; Mangano *et al.*, 2005).

Early cryptogenic focal epilepsy may also start with febrile generalised seizures, which rapidly associate with focal seizures. Distinction can be difficult when the first seizure in DS is focal with or without secondary generalisation. In some patients, an idiopathic focal epilepsy, even Panayiotopoulos syndrome, may be suspected at the very onset due to ictal vomiting (Hino-Fukuyo *et al.*, 2009). These patients will not present atypical absences and myoclonic jerks in the course of the disease but, once more, these are late diagnostic elements. In the first stage, occurrence of alternating hemiclonic seizures and motor seizures affecting different parts of the body is a strong argument against focal epilepsy (Sarisjulis *et al.*, 2000). However, rare patients with focal epilepsy can share clinical features with SMEI and also carry *SCN1A* mutations (Okumura *et al.*, 2007). These cases raise the issue of the diagnostic limits of DS.

Progressive myoclonus epilepsy, particularly late infantile neuronal ceroid-lipofuscinosis (Jansky Bielschowsky) may be evoked in the second year, when myoclonic jerks are prominent and psychomotor development lags. However, this recessive neurometabolic disease runs a more severe course with progressive incessant myoclonus, progressive visual loss, rapid and irreversible language, motor, behavioural and cognitive deterioration, and slowing of EEG background activity. Appropriate neurophysiological, ophthalmologic, biological and molecular testing confirms the diagnosis.

Table II. *A proposed risk score for a screening test (From Hattori* et al.*, 2008). With permission.*

Predictive risk factors	Risk score
Clinical score	
Onset ≤ 7 months	2
Total number of seizures ≥ 5	3
Hemiconvulsions	3
Focal seizure	1
Myoclonic seizure	1
Prolonged seizure	3
Hot-water induced seizure	2
Genetic score	
SCN1A missense mutation	1
SCN1A truncated mutation	2

In the most severe cases, when myoclonic jerks are prominent and a *SCN1A* mutation is absent, a *mitochondrial* defect should also be ruled out by muscle biopsy and a biochemical study of the respiratory chain (Castro-Gago *et al.*, 1997).

Cryptogenic Lennox-Gastaut syndrome (LGS) is virtually excluded by a history of febrile clonic seizures in the first year of life because it begins after one year of age, with a peak between three and eight years. Its characteristics include drop attacks, atypical absences, axial tonic seizures, and specific EEG abnormalities. The latter consist of interictal diffuse slow SWs while awake, which increase during sleep and become poly-SWs, associated with high-voltage rapid rhythms, either subclinical *(Figure 28a)* or accompanied by more or less intense tonic seizures *(Figure 28b)*. LGS is symptomatic in 60% of patients, and can be caused by a high number of genetically determined disorders affecting brain development. The remaining cases are cryptogenic without known genetic aetiology. Some patients with DS exhibit tonic seizures but not during the first two years *(see Figure 14 page 28)*; these are not repeated in clusters and interictal EEGs do not show the typical rapid rhythms. However, a recent paper (Nabbout *et al.*, 2008) reported a sleep EEG pattern resembling that of LGS in five adolescents, of whom three had tonic seizures, which could raise the question of evolution to LGS. The authors agreed that the other characteristics of these patients did not correspond to LGS, and that this feature does not require treatment shift to drugs that could aggravate SMEI.

The onset age is the main element that distinguishes between SMEI and *myoclonic-astatic epilepsy (Doose syndrome)*. In some children with this type of epilepsy, convulsive febrile seizures precede, by several months, non-febrile atonic and myoclonic-astatic seizures which are the hallmark of Doose syndrome, although they rarely start before two years of age. During the course of epilepsy, there are neither partial seizures nor focal features on the EEGs, and the main seizure type is myoclonic-astatic (Guerrini *et al.*, 2005b), whereas isolated drop attacks are unusual in SMEI. Some parents observe sporadic sudden falls in their child, which are not followed by a convulsive seizure. They consider such falls to be due to atonic seizures. However, these have never been documented by polygraphic video-EEG monitoring. They also report episodes of head-nodding during atypical absences. These ictal phenomena are common to EMA and SMEI and do not alter a diagnosis of SMEI.

Other patients with typical SMEI belong to families in which other members present with either febrile seizures or another type of epilepsy and carry a *SCN1A* mutation, in the context of the so-called "GEFS+" (see chapter on genetics).

Mutations in *PCDH19*, the gene encoding protocadherin 19 on the X chromosome, have been described in girls with a clinical picture resembling borderline SMEI who were mutation-negative for *SCN1A*. It will be necessary to study a large number of such patients in order to understand whether mutations of either gene result in overlapping clinical features (see chapter on genetics).

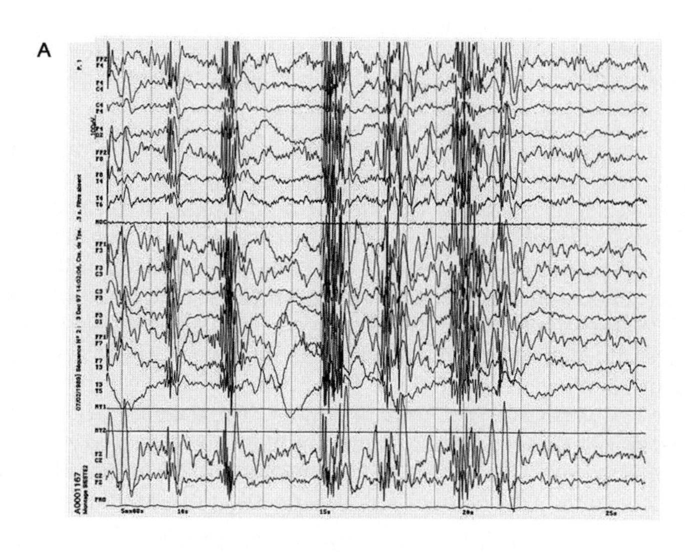

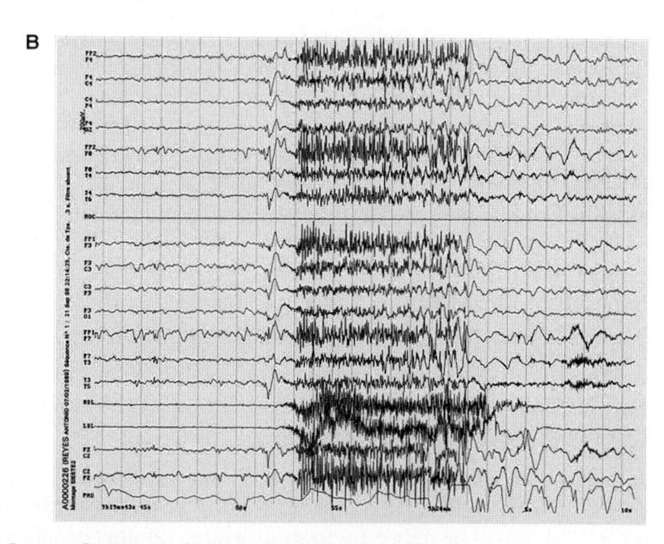

Figure 28a and b. *Lennox-Gastaut syndrome in an eight-year-old boy.*

A: Interictal sleep abnormalities.

Interictal bursts of very high voltage, rapid rhythms, around 20 Hz, during 0.5–1 s, without clinical event, typical for Lennox-Gastaut syndrome.

B: Tonic seizure during slow sleep.

Before the seizure: slow waves, superimposed by a small spike, over the left fronto-temporal area. During the seizure: generalized, slow spike and wave followed by a brief flattening (1 s) preceding a discharge of generalized fast activity of high voltage during 9 s, followed by bifrontal slow waves. EMG shows a bilateral tonic contraction which begins during the flattening and abruptly increases during the rapid discharge, and continues for 1s after the end of the discharge.

RDL: right deltoid muscle; LDL: left deltoid muscle; PNO: pneumogramme.

Diagnostic workup

For an infant aged less than one year, who presents with a first convulsive seizure, either apparently triggered by fever or not, the diagnostic workup is the same as that for a febrile seizure: investigation for an infection, semiologic analysis of the seizure, and history taking for pathological antecedents, family history, and early psychomotor development.

When a second similar seizure occurs shortly thereafter, particular attention should be given to: (1) the semiology of the episode (tonic, clonic, tonic-clonic, generalised from the onset, localised first symptoms, or lateralised on one side); (2) its duration (one minute, five minutes, or more); (3) the degree of temperature (more or less than 38 °C); (4) the possible additional triggering factors (a hot bath); and (5) the effect of acute administration of diazepam or other AEDs (the immediate arrest of the episode or its persistence). If it appears that this seizure was not a simple febrile seizure, an EEG recording while awake and asleep should be obtained, looking for asymmetry, slow background, paroxysmal abnormalities and photosensitivity.

When seizures are repeated, other investigations should be performed. However, the severity of the seizure disorder contrasts with the scarcity of paroxysmal EEG abnormalities, negative aetiological investigations and seemingly normal psychomotor development.

At this point, CT and MRI are usually unrevealing, except for a few cases with dilatation of the cisterna magna or slight diffuse atrophy (Dravet *et al.*, 2005a, b), as is the case for metabolic screening. One must underline the great value of the triggering factors and semiology. The precipitating effect of slight temperature variation, even without true fever, and infections, as well as the lateralisation of the seizure to either side of the body during successive episodes, is characteristic. In this context, genetic testing should be performed for the child, in the knowledge that absence of a *SCN1A* mutation does not preclude diagnosis and should prompt a search for mutations in other genes (Depienne *et al.*, 2009b).

Subsequently, photo- and pattern sensitivity are also frequently observed, including environmental light, which may lead to self-stimulation, sometimes by simple eye closure. Many other stimuli may trigger seizures: hot baths (Awaya *et al.*, 1989), physical exercise (Dravet *et al.*, 2005a, b), noisy environment, or emotion. Such patients have a very high convulsive susceptibility.

During the second year, appearance of other seizure types and EEG abnormalities, as well as retarded development and changes in behaviour which develop into hyperactivity, allow to confirm a diagnosis of SMEI. It is advisable to perform an EEG recording about every six months, with video and polygraphy of muscle activity, when the child is awake, at rest and playing, and during sleep. Such an investigation allows to detect even small myoclonic jerks favoured by movements, and to analyse the correlations between EEG and clinical behaviour of the child. It is also of value to perform repeat cognitive assessments which can detect sectorial deficits (language, visual-perceptive, and visual-motor skills). Neuroimaging should be considered in the first year when the seizures begin. Its results are discussed in a previous chapter. Other ancillary investigations remain normal. The screening test proposed by Hattori *et al.* (2008) although not validated in a prospective fashion, could be useful for general paediatricians who do not have the expertise of a child neurologist. This test is applicable in infants who present with a first febrile seizure in the first year. The main items included in the calculation of a risk score are displayed in *table II* and are in keeping with our own experience.

7. Treatment and Management

"The comprehensive care of a patient with Dravet syndrome encompasses both the 'care' and the 'cure' of the patient, and requires the cooperation between family, doctors, and several other specialised caregivers to search for the attainment of the best quality of life for the patients and their families.... The comprehensive caring must be physician-guided and patient-centred and implies a multidisciplinary approach to be built around the children and caregivers, who need to be guided through the steps of the diagnosis, treatments, and managements of the various comorbidities." (Granata, 2011)

In this chapter, we consider the treatment of epilepsy itself and the management of so-called co-morbidities and related family problems. In spite of recent progress, treatment of DS remains disappointing. This may be explained by the polymorphic nature of seizures and lack of specific drugs for generalised convulsive, focal, absence and myoclonic seizures when they co-occur. A recent meta-analysis of AED therapy for DS underscored the scarcity of controlled studies (Kassai *et al.*, 2008). Pharmacological treatment is the main basis for treatment, although the ketogenic diet is increasingly used. Surgical treatment of epilepsy is contra-indicated, but vagus nerve stimulation is considered an interesting palliative option by some.

Which antiepileptic drugs are useful?

• Among the early AEDs, *Bromides* (Br) were used in Germany and Japan, with significant results against convulsive seizures and status epilepticus (SE). In the study by Oguni *et al.* (1994), five of 22 patients experienced ≥ 75% and two ≥ 50% reduction of their GTCS at 12 months, without noticeable effect on myoclonic seizures. Side effects occurred in 12 children (loss of appetite, drowsiness, ataxia, snoring and skin rash). They gradually disappeared after a slow increase in Br dosage or after reduction of co-medication, but with loss of seizure control in the three patients who had a rash. Recently, Tanabé *et al.* (2008) and Inoue *et al.* (2009) stated that Br was the most widely used and the most effective conventional AED in Japan for convulsive seizures in DS, in the absence of topiramate which is not marketed in Japan.

• *Valproate* (VPA) and *benzodiazepines* (BZDs) offer improvement which is often transitory and is impossible to quantify because no controlled studies have been published. VPA is the first AED usually prescribed and is maintained in many patients, but there is no evidence that its efficacy persists in the long term.

• The most commonly used benzodiazepines are *clonazepam* (CZP) and *clobazam* (CLB). CZP is easy to use because it is available as a solution and doses can be divided during the day. However, in infants, its side effects may be devastating, including drowsiness, hypotonia, ataxia, sialorrhea and upper respiratory tract "drowning". CLB is more popular, but unavailable in solution. Its adverse effects, which often result in irritability and hyperexcitability, can be managed by reducing the dose. In Japan, CLB is included in the group of most efficacious AEDs against SMEI (Tanabe *et al*, 2008; Inoue *et al.*, 2009).

• *Barbiturates* have been largely used without clear improvement and their use is controversial. However, they can be useful in case of convulsive seizures and SE which are resistant to VPA and BZDs.

• *Ethosuximide* (ESM) was used successfully in some patients suffering from countless myoclonic seizures. However, it does not seem to protect against convulsive seizures and its side effects can sometimes be unacceptable: loss of appetite and weight, and withdrawn behaviour.

• *Corticosteroids*, used in cycles of treatment, can be useful in case of repeat SE but do not have long-term efficacy.

• Among the most recent AEDs, several open-label studies show that *Topiramate* (TPM) leads to relatively good control of convulsive and focal seizures (Nieto-Barrera *et al.*, 2000b; Coppola *et al.*, 2002; Villeneuve *et al.*, 2002; Grosso *et al.*, 2005; Kroll-Selger *et al.*, 2006) in spite of side effects. Analysis of these five studies shows that seizure reduction of ≥ 50% occurred in 50 to 85% of patients, of whom 16 to 18% were seizure-free for 11 to 13 months. Maximal daily dosages varied from 9 to 12 mg/kg, with 3 mg/kg being optimal. Slow titration facilitated better tolerance, but side effects were observed in approximately 15% of patients, consisting mainly of anorexia and weight loss, but also behavioural disturbances, emotional and language regression and, more rarely, renal stones. Ceulemans *et al.* (2004) recommended TPM in combination with VPA as the best maintenance treatment, with addition of small doses of BZDs for children who have a history with repeated status epilepticus.

• One recent multicentric, open-label trial evaluated *Levetiracetam* (LEV) in 28 patients, aged three to 23 years, of whom 16 carried a *SCN1A* mutation (Striano *et al.*, 2007b). Follow-up lasted six to 36 months (mean 16.2 ± 13.4). Concomitant medication included 3.6 AEDs; 64.3% of patients were responders for one seizure type (GTCS) with three patients seizure-free, and 39.2% for two seizure types (GTCS and focal or myoclonic seizures) with two patients seizure-free. Four of nine patients (44%) were responders for absences. Three patients had monthly bouts of repeat SE, which disappeared in one. The dosage varied from 750 to 3,000 mg/d (mean 2,016 mg/d) and the target dose was 50-60 mg/Kg/d. Five patients (18%) withdrew from the trial because of side effects which included irritability, cutaneous rash, worsening of myoclonic seizures, and thrombocytopenia, however, the drug was well tolerated in the remaining patients.

• No data are available in Europe for *Zonisamide* (ZNS). In Japan, this drug has been tested for the borderline form with good results if started early (Kanazawa & Shirane, 1999). The authors suggested that ZNS might prevent the appearance of myoclonic seizures. Recently, two reports of retrospective multicentre surveys on DS treatment in Japan considered ZNS as one of the four most effective drugs against convulsive seizures in this syndrome (Tanabe *et al.*, 2008; Inoue *et al.*, 2009).

• Recently, *verapamil*, a voltage-gated calcium channel blocker, was used as add-on therapy in two girls reported by Ianetti *et al.* (2009) with success. It was reported that these two patients experienced seizure-free periods of 13 and 20 months, with improvement in motor and language development in the youngest girl. One open trial is now ongoing in the USA.

• The efficacy of *stiripentol* (STP) was demonstrated in two multicentre randomised, double-blind, placebo-controlled add-on trials (Chiron *et al.*, 2000; Guerrini & Pons, 2000; Guerrini *et al.*, 2002). In the first study (Chiron *et al.*, 2000), 41 patients with SMEI were included, 20 receiving placebo and 21 receiving the active drug at the mean daily dose of 49.3 mg/kg/d. In the STP group, 15 patients (71%) were responders (≥ 50% reduction of clonic and tonic-clonic seizures), including nine who became free of these seizure types, *vs* one (5%) in the placebo group in which none became seizure-free. Plasma concentrations of CLB and nor-clobazam were significantly increased in patients taking STP, compared to baseline, whereas concentrations of hydroxynorclobazam were significantly decreased. This observation was explained by the study of Giraud *et al.* (2006) showing that STP inhibits the formation of NCLB from CLB and even more strongly the formation of hydroxynorclobazam from NCLB.

Moderate side effects occurred in all STP-treated patients (drowsiness, loss of appetite, and loss of weight) *vs* five (25%) on placebo, although the side effects disappeared when the doses of the co-medication (VPA, CLB) were decreased in 17 of the 21 cases. These findings were confirmed by an Italian study (Guerrini & Pons, 2000; Guerrini *et al.*, 2000) conducted with a similar design and protocol; 67% of patients on STP *vs* 9% of those on placebo met the response criteria. Kassai *et al.* (2008) performed a meta-analysis of these two trials and reported odds ratio of response to STP relative to placebo of 32 (CI: 6.2, 161) with an overall seizure rate reduction of 70% (93%; 47%) associated with STP.

The long-term efficacy and safety of STP were reported in another study (Than *et al.*, 2002). In 46 patients, seizure frequency and duration were significantly reduced, as was the number of convulsive SE during a median follow-up of three years. Ten patients (22%) dramatically improved and episodes of SE disappeared. Twenty patients (43%) moderately improved, mainly as a result of the reduction of seizure duration and the number of episodes of convulsive SE. Four (9%) had no response and efficacy could not be evaluated in 12, mainly because of adverse effects. Loss of appetite and weight prevented increasing the dose to 50 mg/kg/d in patients older than 12 years.

In Japan, Inoue *et al.* (2009) performed an open-label multicentre add-on study of STP in 25 patients with DS, divided into two groups according to age; 17 between one and eight year old (younger group: Y) and eight between 13 and 22 year old (older group: E). Results were almost comparable to those obtained in the two European studies with ≥ 50% seizure reduction in 61%, of whom two were seizure-free. Duration of GTCS was reduced, and SE and seizure clusters were less frequent. In addition, efficacy and tolerability were similar in older compared to younger patients. It is noteworthy that STP was always combined with VPA, but also with several other AEDs, and a more efficacious combination was not identified. Among the responders, some were treated with CLB and also had defective activity of CYP2C19; the enzyme that metabolizes NCLB. This observation indicates that the beneficial effects of STP are not explained by a simple pharmacokinetic interaction. Other responders did not receive CLB, which indicates that STP might be effective on its own.

Although the efficacy of STP was demonstrated in combination with VPA and CLB in the two controlled trials, a direct antiepileptic effect of STP is likely, as suggested by the Japanese study (Inoue *et al.*, 2009) as well as anecdotal use in some patients. Several authors also came to the conclusion that STP is an "anticonvulsant per se" (Chiron & Dulac, 2011; Prunetti & Perucca, 2011).

This hypothesis is strongly supported by a series of pharmacological experiments by Fisher (2009, 2011a,b) showing that (i) STP acts as a direct allosteric modulator of the GABA receptor at a site distinct from many commonly used anti-convulsant, sedative and anxiolytic drugs; (ii) the δ-containing receptors are insensitive to modulation by benzodiazepines but sensitive to STP. The authors therefore suggested that (i) STP would enhance activity of both synaptic and extrasynaptic populations of $GABA_A$ receptors; (ii) polytherapy is expected to increase the maximum effect beyond that of either drug alone; (iii) STP can show efficacy in patient populations that are pharmacoresistant to benzodiazepines; and STP is a rational choice for polytherapy with benzodiazepine agonists.

On the whole, STP has proven useful in decreasing the frequency and duration of convulsive seizures and the number of episodes of SE. However, this drug has not yet been properly evaluated for the remaining seizure types, including photosensitive seizures.

Which antiepileptic drugs should be avoided?

Any AED can have a paradoxical effect by exacerbating epileptic seizures in any type of epilepsy, and DS is no exception. Two AEDs in particular, *carbamazepine* (CBZ) and *lamotrigine* (LTG), have been shown to bear the potential to aggravate seizures in most patients.

For CBZ, seizure aggravation was reported in at least three reports (Horn *et al.*, 1986; Wakai *et al.*, 1996b; Wang *et al.*, 1996).

An aggravating effect of LTG was demonstrated by Guerrini *et al.* (1998). In this report, LTG induced seizure worsening in 17 of 21 patients (80%), no change in three, and improvement in one. Worsening was observed mainly in convulsive and myoclonic seizures. It appeared clearly within three months in most patients but occasionally had an insidious course, also enhanced by slow titration of the drug. These findings were confirmed by Wallace (1998).

The aggravating effects of *phenytoin* (PHT) were reported anecdotally. Two authors reported paroxysmal movement disorders in patients with DS treated by polytherapy, including PHT (Saito *et al.*, 2001; Ohtsuka *et al.*, 2003). All patients presented with frequent seizures and the paroxysmal movements appeared after the PHT dosage was increased, without additional signs of toxicity. This side effect of PHT is well known in patients with severe epilepsy and mental impairment (Dravet *et al.*, 1980, 1983; Zaatreh *et al.*, 2001). No clear information is available regarding possible worsening of seizures.

The three AEDs mentioned above are not similar but share a common mechanism of action which involves the use-dependent inhibition of sodium channels necessary for the "firing" of action potentials, responsible for convulsive seizures. This property might explain their ability to increase seizures when epilepsy is caused by a sodium channelopathy. AED-induced seizure worsening does not appear in all patients and might also be influenced by age. In some older patients taking polytherapies, including PHT, CBZ or LTG, attempts at drug withdrawal were followed by aggravation of epilepsy.

In infants and children, *Vigabatrin* should be avoided as it has the potential to increase the frequency of myoclonic seizures. However, in older patients, this drug may be effective against convulsive and focal seizures.

ALTERNATIVE TREATMENTS

Ketogenic diet

It was noted early in history that fasting could be used for the treatment of epilepsy. Descriptions of dietary restriction for many diseases, including epilepsy, date back to the time of Hippocrates and are mentioned in the New Testament.

The ketogenic diet (KD) is a non-pharmacological treatment which was first developed in the US for intractable childhood seizures in the 1920s, when a faith healer and an osteopathic physician advocated the use of fasting and prayer in a boy with seizures (Swink *et al.*, 1997, cited by Hartmann & Vining, 2007). At that time, few AEDs were available, and the KD was put aside following the discovery of phenytoin in 1938. However, in spite of more recently introduced AEDs, many childhood epilepsies remain uncontrolled and recent interest in the KD was precipitated by the treatment of a child at the Johns Hopkins Hospital, about 15 years ago, largely publicised by a movie.

The principle of the KD was based on the biology of starvation, where fat metabolism becomes a major energy source, replacing glucose and other carbohydrates. It was hypothesized that a high fat diet could mimic ketosis produced by fasting. However, the mechanism by which ketone bodies exert an anticonvulsive effect remains unexplained, in spite of modern research, and proposed mechanisms are likely to emerge in the near future.

The KD is high in fat content and low in protein and carbohydrate. The diet is calculated based on the ratio of grams of fats to grams of proteins plus carbohydrates. The ratio is commonly 4 g of fats to 1 g of proteins plus carbohydrates (4:1). This means that 90% of the energy comes from fat and 10% from protein and carbohydrate combined. Sometimes, it is necessary to recommend the KD at a lower ratio in order to increase protein or carbohydrate intake.

The modalities of the diet, which have been applied in many different ways, are not discussed here. Consensus papers have been published by panels of experts (Kossof *et al.*, 2009; Veggiotti *et al.*, 2011). Several prerequisites are important before initiating the diet. Some metabolic disorders, including disorders of fatty acid transport, β oxidation and some mitochondrial cytopathies, are aggravated by KD, and must be ruled out for children who are candidates for this diet. As the restricting diet has consequences on general health and growth, it must be conducted by a multidisciplinary team, comprising child neurologist, nutritionist, endocrinologist, dietician, and psychologist.

The KD requires a strict application and therefore a good comprehension of the regimen by the parents, as well as close collaboration between family, doctors and dieticians.

The KD has been reported to benefit children with DS in several papers. In a series of 24 patients treated with KD in Argentina (Caraballo, 2011) and followed for a minimum of two years, 16 (66.6%) remained on the diet after achieving a significant improvement; seizure freedom was reported in two, a 75-99% decrease in seizures in ten, and a 50-74% decrease in four. No complications were reported in this group. Six patients were off the diet for more than two years. Three had improved with just sporadic seizures and three had relapsed. Of the remaining eight patients, three did not tolerate the diet, which was interrupted soon after the start (severe vomiting) and five did not continue the diet because of lack of efficacy.

Korff *et al.* (2007) reported positive results in four of six patients. Dressler *et al.* (2010) retrospectively studied 50 children with drug-resistant epilepsies treated by KD between 1999 and 2008. Eight patients (16%) suffered from genetically-confirmed DS. Responders were those patients presenting with ≥ 50% reduction in seizure frequency. In the whole series, 50% were responders: 4/9 with infantile spasms, 2/4 with LGS, and 5/8 with DS. The latter were not identified in the analysis of the results. For all patients, favourable predicting factors were a short duration of epilepsy before starting the KD and the presence of GTCS. Only few side effects were observed in this population, which never led to discontinuation of the diet and were significantly associated with TPM and VPA as co-medication.

Nabbout *et al.* (2011) tested the efficacy of the KD in 15 patients with partial response to AEDs including STP. They considered only seizures with a clonic component (generalized, unilateral or focal) and defined the responders as those patients with a decrease of seizure frequency ≥ 75%. Fifty percent of patients were responders at three and six months and 40% at nine months. All responders had also improvement in attention and reduced hyperactivity, as confirmed by Conners and Achenbach scales.

Immunotherapy

Only one small study has focused on the immunological aspects of SMEI, without reaching definite conclusions (Nieto *et al.*, 2000). However, considering the sensitivity to infections and their role in triggering seizures, we personally administered *immunoglobulins* to some patients with relative success. Interesting results have been reported by Nieto-Barrera *et al.* (1995).

Vagus nerve stimulation

This palliative treatment is still in evaluation for DS but does not seem to be very efficacious. Zamponi *et al.* (2010) applied this procedure to eight patients with DS, all carrying a *SCN1A* mutation. Implantation was performed in childhood and adolescence (5-13 years) except in one patient, at 25 years. All patients, but one, exhibited GTCS, four had myoclonic seizures, and one had complex partial seizures only. Vagus nerve stimulation (VNS) produced a mean seizure rate reduction of 12% at three months, 6% at six months, and 31% at twelve months. The maximum reduction rate was 61% in a single patient, around 50% in three, 33% in one and zero in three. The authors could not draw any conclusion with regards to improvement of seizure types and no improvement was obtained in patients who had suffered episodes of status epilepticus. After one year of VNS, cognitive level was unchanged but improvement in adapting behaviour and communication was observed, with better quality of life in one.

Deep brain stimulation

Deep brain stimulation (DBS) is an alternative treatment for medically refractory epilepsies which cannot be cured by epilepsy surgery. This method is still under development and has been applied to only three patients with DS (Chabardès *et al.*, 2002; Andrade *et al.*, 2010). To summarise, the three patients presented with a high number of generalised tonic-clonic seizures (60 and 15 per month, respectively), associated with sporadic myoclonic jerks in one. One patient (Chabardès *et al.*, 2002), stimulated in the subthalamic nucleus, was a moderate responder with a mean seizure frequency reduction of 41.5%, which was considered to be insufficient and the battery was removed. The two remaining patients (Andrade *et al.*, 2010) were implanted in the anterior thalamus. One proved to be a good responder with a mean seizure frequency reduction of 81%, which persisted for ten years, without change in myoclonic jerks. The second patient did not experience a decrease in seizure frequency during the five years of stimulation. No conclusion may be drawn from these few cases and further studies are needed to better understand the networks implicated in the seizures of DS and the mechanisms of the DBS itself.

When to start continuous treatment and how to conduct it?

After one isolated febrile or afebrile seizure in an infant aged less than one year, rectal diazepam should be prescribed in order to prevent a possible subsequent seizure lasting for longer than a few minutes. It is reasonable to consider SMEI as a possible diagnosis:

- if two additional seizures, especially when lateralised, occur after a short interval (days or weeks) without a temperature spike;
- if a seizure has either evolved to SE or proven to be resistant to rectal injection;
- if workup for symptomatic seizures is negative;
- if other seizure types (focal, myoclonic) appear;
- if spontaneous or light-induced epileptic EEG abnormalities appear;
- even if convulsive seizures are not frequently repeated at the onset.

At this point, a continuous treatment should be initiated *(Figure 29)*.

Pharmacological treatment

Monotherapy with VPA is the first classical option. It is usually well tolerated but the risk of hepatic failure dictates the necessity to monitor VPA plasma levels and biological constants when the infant has repeated vomiting. If other seizures occur, in spite of average VPA plasma levels, two options may be deemed. The first is to combine VPA, CLB and STP, which is the best drug combination in most patients, particularly to avoid early status epilepticus and their presumed impact on cognitive outcome (Chiron, 2011).

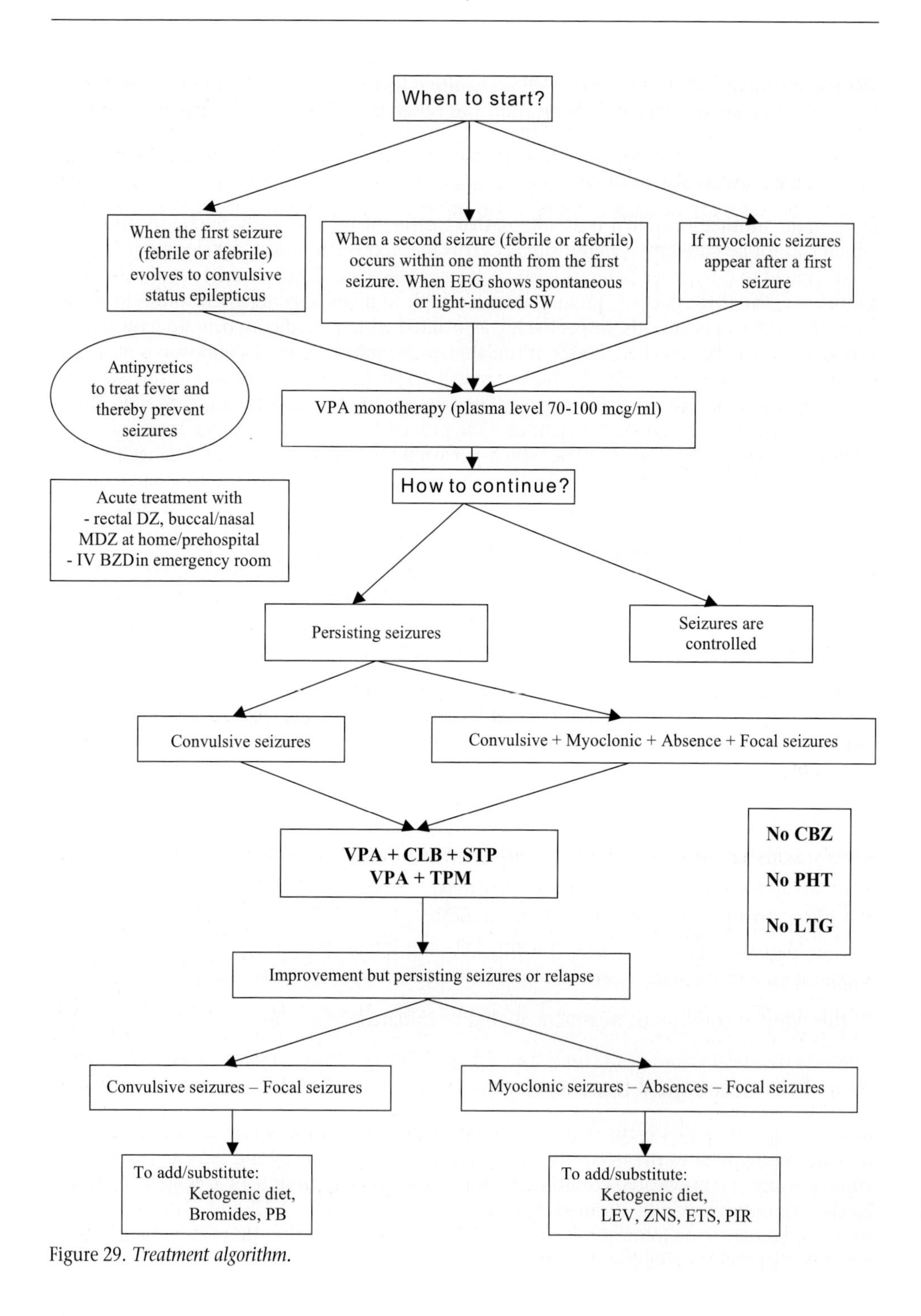

Figure 29. *Treatment algorithm.*

The second is to combine VPA and TPM, particularly in countries where STP is not available. In this case, particular attention must be given to the development and alertness of the infant, which could be negatively influenced by TPM. VPA and potassium bromide (KBr) is an alternative second choice combination. In most patients, complete control is never reached and the possible initial positive effect does not last more than weeks or months. Thus, subsequent changes in AEDs are necessary, using substitution rather than addition, in order to avoid heavy polytherapies. As already mentioned, CZP, ZNS, and LEV, in various combinations, including or not STP, can be prescribed. Some authors propose to limit the use of BZDs, when possible, because of their side effects (Ceulemans *et al.*, 2004) and when chronic treatment is not well tolerated, their punctual administration is helpful.

When *atypical absences and myoclonic seizures* are extremely frequent, ETS may be particularly effective. We have successfully used *Piracetam* (PIR) at high doses in some cases but, we have also observed poor tolerance in other cases.

Other therapeutic measures

Ketogenic diet

The role of the KD is difficult to define. It can be offered early in the course of the disease when the first AEDs are ineffective or poorly tolerated, even in the first year. Most authors suggest that the best results of the KD are obtained early after onset of the epilepsy (Dressler *et al.*, 2010). The diet can also be proposed to patients with repeated bouts of status epilepticus at any age.

In any case, it is recommended not to wait until the patient has already received all possible medications, keeping in mind that the diet is easier to apply in young children than adolescents and that full cooperation between the family, neuropaediatrician and dietician is mandatory.

Fever

Clearly, body temperature should be monitored regularly. During the first months, parents quickly learn the range of temperature that puts their child "at risk" and when they must administer an antipyretic drug. Oral or rectal paracetamol (acetaminophen) is the most widely used drug. Interactions with other drugs must be considered, especially when the child also receives VPA. A reversible acute hepatic impairment was reported in five children with SMEI when acetaminophen was added to their therapy because they were febrile and presented with status epilepticus (two patients), postictal sopor (one patient), or respiratory infection (two patients). The associated drugs were VPA and TPM in four (Nicolai *et al.*, 2008), and VPA, STP and CLB in one (Goorhuis *et al.*, 2008). However, these cases are exceptional when compared to the high number of patients receiving both VPA and acetaminophen. Nishri *et al.* (2010) reported a patient carrying a *SCN1A* mutation who developed hepatic coma after febrile status epilepticus treated with BZD, PHT, PB and acetaminophen. Muscle biopsy showed "mitochondrial disfunction" but the authors did not find a satisfactory explanation for the association of SMEI and muscle biopsy findings, in the absence of a *POLG1* mutation.

Acetaminophen should be used in case of fever, without exceeding the recommended doses and with hepatic enzyme monitoring.

Prevention of body temperature increase is recommended by avoiding hot environmental conditions, hot baths, maintaining good hydration, providing ice and cold liquids in the summer, and moderating physical activity. Special "cooling" clothes, available on the internet, can help to avoid temperature increase.

Photo- and pattern sensitivity

Photo- and pattern sensitivity, variably associated with self-stimulation, are extremely drug-resistant and can produce long-lasting obtundation and myoclonic status, as well as clonic seizures.

Precaution is required when watching television, for example: the use of a television screen 100 or 120 Hz, watching at a distance from the screen, and a lightened room, however, often these preventive measures are not sufficient. Outdoor, wearing sunglasses is recommended but also not sufficient.

Several studies have demonstrated that photosensitivity in epilepsy is not homogeneous and cannot be controlled by the use of any commercially available blue lens (Takahashi & Tsukahara, 1992; Capovilla *et al.*, 2006). Z1 lenses seem to be particularly effective, causing the photoparoxysmal response to IPS to disappear in 75.9% of patients and decrease in 17.9%.

Takahashi *et al.* (1995) accurately studied photosensitivity and self-induction of seizures in a patient with DS. These authors hypothesised that self-induction might have wavelength specificity and absorption by appropriate optical filters may reduce photosensitivity and exert an inhibitory effect on the manœuvre used by the child, such as forced eye closure and waving hand movements. Continuously wearing these specific lenses gradually decreased the occurrence of self-stimulation.

Given these data, we strongly recommend the prescription of Z1 lenses, or equivalent in terms of optical characteristics, to children who have pronounced sensitivity to daylight, *a fortiori*, to those who engage in self-stimulation. It is important to optimally adapt the glasses to each patient in order to intercept all the light reaching the eyes, even laterally *(see photos in Annex 3)*.

Unfortunately, *pattern sensitivity* is not inhibited by these lenses in the same way, but can be attenuated in some. Based on the observation that monocular light and pattern stimulation fail to provoke epileptic discharges, glasses masking one eye are more efficacious but cannot be worn continuously.

Other triggering factors should be avoided such as intense emotional situations and other individual factors.

How to treat seizures and status epilepticus

Clonic and tonic-clonic seizures

Clonic and tonic-clonic seizures do not require acute treatment when brief and isolated. One simple protective measure against ictal respiratory failure during sleep is to remove large pillows, fluffy animals or soft toys from the bed. When seizures last more than five minutes (potential status epilepticus), or when they recur at short intervals, it is preferable to interrupt them in order to reduce the risk of status epilepticus. We consider short intervals those in between several seizures that recur during the same day or the same night. Seizures can be brief but repeated in clusters, for example: three episodes in one hour, with or without provoking factors. When the interval between two seizures is less than half an hour or when it progressively shortens, the transition to status epilepticus may be imminent.

Using rectal diazepam can prevent the transition of a long seizure to status. This procedure remains the most widely used by parents and professional caregivers whatever the epileptic syndrome, and is reliable for infants and young children, although difficult to apply in adolescents and adults. Buccal or nasal administration of midazolam solution has recently been demonstrated to provide the same results. Several studies have compared efficacy and safety of the two compounds. A meta-analysis of six studies, comprising 774 subjects presenting with an epileptic seizure lasting more than five minutes, has confirmed that non-intravenous midazolam, compared to non-intravenous or intravenous diazepam, was safe and effective (Mc Mullan *et al.*, 2010). Unfortunately, in some countries, midazolam is not available for buccal/nasal administration, being restricted to intravenous route and only for hospital use. Other benzodiazepines (clonazepam, lorazepam) were not studied but probably could be efficacious when used orally. Thus, in practice, two procedures are possible: either rectal diazepam or buccal/nasal midazolam or, alternatively, buccal lorazepam and clonazepam. As the absorption is sublingual, swallowing is not required.

However, patients with DS, who often experience periods of worsening with numerous seizures, are at risk of receiving too many doses of BZD with deleterious side effects (drowsiness, gait imbalance, irritability, poor attention and dribbling with increased risk of an ingestis) which need to be carefully weighed against the risks inherent in seizure occurrence. With time, parents and caregivers become aware of the usual course of seizures and know when a cluster will stop spontaneously or evolve into status.

Status epilepticus can occur because no treatment was applied or in spite of treatment. No guidelines have been established for the treatment of status epilepticus in DS, although the protocols for status epilepticus in children are reliable, based on the use of intravenous benzodiazepines (mainly midazolam, lorazepam and clonazepam), phenytoin and fosphenytoin, valproate, barbiturates, and more rarely, anaesthetics and propofol. Recently, levetiracetam was added to this armamentarium (Abend *et al.*, 2010), however, although the use of this drug has produced interesting results in some patients, further studies are needed to evaluate its usefulness.

Attention must be drawn to avoiding accumulation of high doses of AEDs which can induce metabolic and haemodynamic failure. This is especially important for barbiturates, which require careful monitoring of the plasma levels to avoid serious complications (Chipaux *et al.*, 2010).

The role of barbiturates is unclear. Tanabe *et al.* (2008) reported that in Japan, barbiturates are often considered to be the most effective drugs. Dooley *et al.* (1995) reported on two Canadian children who were successfully treated with pentobarbital on multiple occasions, through a subcutaneous permanent central line. Barbiturates should be used with caution and only in the hospital, with monitoring of plasma levels.

In DS, fever, respiratory infections, vaccinations, and treatment changes are the most frequent causes of status epilepticus and must be systematically investigated. Acute encephalopathy associated with influenza and other viral infections, characterised by febrile status epilepticus followed by coma and, sometimes, multi-organ failure, was reported in one child (Takayanagi *et al.*, 2010). This encephalopathy, which can be lethal or lead to severe sequelae, is more frequent in Japan than in other countries (Amin *et al.*, 2008).

Other seizure types

Atypical absences, myoclonic seizures and focal seizures can have a negative impact on behaviour and learning when they are frequently repeated and oral/rectal/nasal BZD may be used on occasion. These seizures can evolve into status too. In this case, acute treatment must be applied because of the risk of superimposed GTCS. Usually, non-convulsive status is more responsive to treatment than convulsive status.

To summarise, since no single AED or AED combination has been demonstrated to completely control seizures, it is preferable to avoid heavy polytherapies which have a deleterious effect on behaviour and learning. The aim of the treatment should not be to achieve complete seizure remission but to decrease frequency and duration while favouring cognitive development. Avoiding triggering factors when possible decreases the risk for seizures. In case of prolonged seizures, every family should be given a plan for emergency treatment to be applied before hospital admission, and subsequently in the emergency room, with precise timing and dosing of the drugs. Some families request an oxygen delivery device at home, but this is not really effective unless an aspirator is also available to clean the upper respiratory tract of secretions.

Parents often ask if gene therapy and the use of stem cells should be considered. Several areas of experimental research are ongoing in order to answer this question (Naegele *et al.*, 2010), particularly concerning read-through drugs for nonsense mutations (Delgado-Escueta & Bourgeois, 2008). These studies create reasonable hope for the future, but until now, no procedure has been identified that could be applied in the short term to patients.

What about compulsory vaccinations?

An association between vaccination and initial seizures in DS has been previously reported (Dravet *et al.*, 1982; Nieto Barrera *et al.*, 2000a; Caraballo & Fejerman, 2006). This observation is not surprising since the first year of life is also the time when the first legal vaccinations are performed. Since coincidence between seizures and vaccination is often observed, parents and some doctors tend to conclude that a causal relationship exists between the two events. This situation is similar to that of infants with West syndrome, since infantile spasms also begin in the first year of life. Clearly, coincidence is insufficient to support this hypothesis which was recently discarded in scientific studies. In the literature, cases of "vaccine encephalopathies" have been reported, consisting of epileptic seizures and developmental regression occurring in the days following vaccination, mainly pertussis vaccination, in previously healthy infants. Berkovic *et al.* (2006) retrospectively analyzed 14 patients with alleged vaccine encephalopathy in whom the first seizure occurred within 72 hours of vaccination. A specific epilepsy syndrome was diagnosed in all cases: DS in 12 (11 with a *SCN1A* mutation) and LGS in two (without *SCN1A* mutation). These findings indicate that vaccination may trigger epileptic seizures in infants who are susceptible but is not, by itself, the cause of epilepsy. The mechanism at stake remains unknown since post-vaccine seizures can occur without fever. Tro-Baumann *et al.* (2011) investigated 70 patients with DS and *SCN1A* mutation in order to clarify the frequency of these seizures. They identified 19 patients (27%) who had 34 seizures within 72 hours following vaccination (6-11 days for attenuated vaccines). The vast majority of seizures (79%) were related to diphtheria-tetanos-pertussis immunisation in tri-, penta-, and hexavalent, as well as other, combinations. One third of seizures was not associated with fever. Eight patients experienced prolonged seizures or status, which were followed by subsequent similar episodes remotly from vaccination. In 11 patients, the vaccination-related seizures were the first ictal episodes to be reported, a finding similar to previous reports (Nieto Barrera *et al.*, 2000a; Caraballo & Fejerman, 2006). The authors suggested to perform genetic screening in infants with this clinical presentation, in order to improve early diagnosis and treatment of DS.

In spite of the recognized association between vaccination and seizure occurrence in a subset of infants with DS, it is proven that vaccines are only a triggering and not a causative factor. Thus, vaccinations should be performed in these patients, because infectious diseases can be serious and also provoke seizures, as demonstrated by Tanabe *et al.* (2004). These authors found the rate of neurological complications (status, encephalopathy) to be higher ($p < 0.0001$) during naturally contracted measles, rubella, mumps, and influenza (63%) than after vaccination (7.2%). McIntosh *et al.* (2010) compared outcome in two groups of patients; those with a first seizure close to vaccination and those with a first seizure apparently unrelated to vaccination. They found no differences in intellectual outcome, subsequent seizure types or genetic mutation between the two groups.

Although there are no true preventive measures, we recommend that a vaccine should not be injected when the child is ill or febrile and antipyretics should be administered before and after the vaccination, in combination with BZDs over a period of a week.

How to manage miscellaneous problems

As children with DS present with multiple problems, they need to be cared for not only by a neuropaediatrician, but also by other specialists according to their individual clinical characteristics.

Motor impairment can be attenuated by physiotherapy and psychomotricity.

Treatment for *cyphoscoliosis* and foot deformities depends on the orthopaedist, keeping in mind there is no definite treatment and results of surgery are variable. Orthopaedic problems are particularly worrying in adult patients.

Feeding difficulties and failure to thrive are frequent and can require counselling with a nutritionist. When chewing/swallowing difficulties and lack of appetite evolve to refusal of food, oral feeding becomes inadequate and very time-consuming. At this point, gastrostomy tube (G-tube) placement, usually by percutaneous endoscopic gastrostomy (PEG), may be considered, but this procedure should remain exceptional because complications can occur. Training of families and caregivers is important for care. In our experience, we encountered this situation only twice. Confronted with growth failure, an endocrinologist should be consulted.

Sleep disorders can be induced by the timing of seizures. Nocturnal seizures are followed by daytime drowsiness, whereas diurnal seizures with postictal sleep, especially in late afternoon, lead to a subsequent delay in falling asleep. Children may also wake up during the night. Prescription of melatonin or sleep-inducers is helpful.

Cognitive impairment and behavioural disorders.

As soon as the diagnosis of DS is confirmed, it is advised to regularly assess the development of the infant or child. Periodic cognitive evaluations allow for a better understanding of the factors responsible for the delayed milestones and the respective roles of seizures and AEDs.

An infant with DS is at risk of becoming a disabled person and it is possible to decrease the degree of this handicap by offering him/her a good environment with appropriate educative and rehabilitative methods (psychomotricity, speech therapy, and ergotherapy). Socialisation is important but difficult. Integration in school depends on the local resources and on the cooperation of the teachers. If possible, classes for children with special needs are to be preferred. Later on, most adolescent and adult patients should attend specialised institutions, although few may benefit from sheltered working structures.

Management of behavioural disturbances is difficult and psychological support by a specialised team can help the patients and their families. Poor comprehension and poor verbal communication largely contribute to the deterioration of social relationships with other children, leading to withdrawal, but rarely to aggressiveness. These problems often worsen in adolescence, especially in patients with only slight or mild cognitive impairment who become aware of their being different and do not accept it. Pharmacological treatment is not appropriate, except in the case of psychiatric episodes, which are infrequent. Conversely, physicians should be aware of the possible exacerbation of pathological behaviours by some AEDs (LEV, ZNS, TPM, BZDs, *etc.*)

How to help families

Families and caregivers of patients suffering from such a devastating form of epilepsy should be helped by doctors, professionals and other people.

Support should start from the time of diagnosis. However, whether it is actually beneficial for families to be told of the diagnosis immediately following the first ictal episodes, is a major dilemma. Due to genetic advances, very early molecular diagnosis is now possible in most patients. This allows for the most appropriate drugs to be used, avoiding therapeutic errors, "cutting" status epilepticus, and early detection of developmental delay and planning the most appropriate educational measures. When parents plan for another pregnancy, early diagnosis also enables the risk for the future child being affected to be assessed. However, explaining DS to parents when they do not have any knowledge of an epileptic disease and when their baby is still healthy and developing well, may lead to depressive reactions, and sometimes, to denial of the diagnosis. Doctors should try to access the individual situations of parents. Because of their anxiety, some parents do not ask for much information. In these cases, doctors might prefer to postpone the announcement until the parents become aware of something wrong and question doctors on their own.

In any case, it is important to clearly illustrate treatment options, give written instructions on how to behave in case of a seizure (see above), answer questions and create a trustworthy relationship. At the onset, frequent medical consultations should reassure parents. Sometimes it is easier for parents to express their concerns with a nurse.

When the diagnosis is well established and the parents are informed, a discussion is advised on how to monitor the child's development and propose support by a specialised team to realise the best conditions to favour learning. Such a process can also help the family to organise itself, keeping in mind that siblings may feel neglected when the parents devote most of their time and attention to the affected child. The parental couple can experience social isolation as other family members are often frightened by the idea of dealing with a child with frequent seizures. In some countries, hospitals can offer periods of respite to the family, the patient being cared by nurses for one or several days, but this system is rarely available (Nolan *et al.*, 2006, 2008). For adolescents and adults, specialised institutions may provide these respite periods. At the very least, it is essential that parents and siblings are given the possibility to express their difficulties to doctors and other caregivers and being heard, possibly through psychological support.

Recently, family associations have rapidly grown in different countries, the largest being the IDEA League, which provides an internet discussion forum and meetings. Many families find this initiative invaluable for communicating with others who face similar problems. These associations also support research of the disease and organise successful fundraising events. Those involved have become "spokesmen" for all the patients and families by expressing their grief and expectations, not only to doctors who are insufficiently informed on this particular type of epilepsy, but also to society and government representatives (Skluzacek *et al.*, 2011).

8. Long Term Outcome

Available knowledge indicates that SMEI is always associated with an unfavourable outcome. All patients are reported to have persistent seizures and be cognitively impaired, often severely. Several authors have published series of patients followed to adolescence (Giovanardi Rossi *et al.*, 1991; Yakoub *et al.*, 1992; Ohki *et al.*, 1997; Fontana *et al.*, 2004; Caraballo & Fejerman, 2006), but only three series included patients older than 20 years (Jansen *et al.*, 2006; Dravet *et al.*, 2009; Akiyama *et al.*, 2010; Genton *et al.*, 2011). The number of patients, their age and genetic findings are summarised in *Table III.*

This chapter is mainly based on the results of these studies. In our series, some of the patient information at last follow-up was obtained by correspondence or telephone calls.

Seizures

Whatever the type, seizures are extremely resistant to any kind of treatment during the first years, requiring numerous hospitalisations. Later on, partial seizures, myoclonic seizures and atypical absences tend to disappear but convulsive seizures persist, occurring mainly during night-time sleep. They can be repeated during the same night, especially in the case of fever, and may be preceded by myoclonic jerks.

Table III. *Long-term studies in the literature.*

Study	Patient number			Ages (years)			Mutation			
	Total	Typical form	Borderline form	Range	Mean	Median	SCN1A	GABRG2	None	Not tested
Jansen *et al.*, 2006	14	8	6	18-47	26	23	10	1	3	
Dravet *et al.*, 2009	24	23	1	18-47	29	28	6		5	13
Akiyama *et al.*, 2010	31	14	17	18-43	24	22	23		6	2

The period of very active epilepsy varies from one child to another, sometimes extending up to the age of 12-13 years. Likewise Ohki *et al.* (1997), we found no homogeneous age of disappearance of myoclonic jerks, atypical absences or partial seizures. However, in two very long-term studies, seven patients were reported to become seizure-free for at least one year and up to five years *(Table IV)*. In two patients, such prolonged remission was obtained after addition of topiramate.

In the remaining patients, the frequency of convulsive seizures progressively decreased. At the end of follow-up, the frequency of seizures was reported to be between one and twelve per year and often in clusters by Dravet *et al.* (2009) and between one and ten per year by Akiyama et al. (2010). In our experience, some patients suffered recurrent periods of worsening during adolescence and early adulthood without recognisable triggering factors. Akiyama *et al.* (2010) also found periods of increasing frequency in some young adults, although the overall trend was towards a decrease after the age of 25 years.

Convulsive status epilepticus was no longer observed after the age of ten by Akiyama *et al.* (2010), but in our series still occurred between the ages of 24 and 28 years. We also observed obtundation status in some patients (Genton *et al.*, 2011). The other seizure types often disappeared *(Table V)*.

Fever and infections were triggering factors for only half of the cases in our series and in one third in the study of Akiyama *et al.* (2010).

Table IV. *Seizure-free patients at follow-up.*

Study	Patients	Seizure free	Ages	Duration	Treatment
Jansen *et al.*, 2006	14	0			
Dravet *et al.*, 2009	24	2	26 to 31 28 to 30	5 years 2 years	TPM added TPM added
Akiyama *et al.*, 2010	31	5	27 to 30 26 to 29 19 to 21 19 to 21 19 to 20	3 years 3 years 2 years 2 years 1 year	? ? ? ? ?

Table V. *Seizure types at long-term followu-up.*

Study	Patients	GCS	Convulsive status	Obtundation status	Atypical absences	Myoclonic seizures	Focal seizures	Other
Jansen *et al.*, 2006	14	14	NA	NA	4	2	7	1 atonic seizure
Dravet*et al.*, 2009	24	22	3	4	6	2	1	
Akiyama *et al.*, 2010	21	25	None	2	2	2	8	

GCS: generalized convulsive; NA: not available.

Photo- and pattern sensitivity are difficult to study as they are not constant in the same patient during follow-up, however, all authors have reported a tendency of visual-sensitivity to disappear in adolescence and adulthood. In the series reported by Akiyama *et al.* (2010), seven patients had photo- or pattern sensitivity during childhood, which was present in only one patient after the age of 31. Genton *et al.* (2011) reported a 21-year-old patient who still presented photosensitivity and self-stimulation.

EEG

No information on EEG was provided by Jansen *et al.* (2006). In our series, several EEG recordings were performed during adulthood although not on a regular basis and EEG findings observed at different times in adulthood are presented below. Akiyama *et al.* (2010) reported EEG findings only in the last year of follow-up for their adult patients. These EEG data are summarised in *table VI.*

Background activity fluctuates, depending on the number and severity of seizures. *Background activity* remained normal, and an occipital alpha rhythm was present in around one third of cases for Dravet *et al.* (2009) and in two thirds for Akiyama *et al.* (2010). A peculiar strong increase of theta activity in the central regions and vertex, elicited by eye closure is often observed (Bureau & Dalla Bernardina, 2011). This activity is particularly enhanced in patients showing an intense tremor with deterioration of motor abilities.

Interictal paroxysmal EEG abnormalities can disappear completely or become sporadic. They are represented by focal and multifocal spikes, SWs and sharp waves, rarely associated with generalised SWs. Focal *abnormalities* often appear only during sleep. The cyclic organisation of sleep remained normal in 70% of the patients in whom it was assessed. In the remaining cases, although the sleep architecture was not preserved, distinction between REM and nREM sleep was still possible.

Table VI. *Interictal EEG in adult patients.*

EEG characteristics	Akiyama *et al.*, 2010 31 pts	Dravet *et al.*, 2009 24 pts	Total 55 pts
Background			
subnormal	20	8	28
slow	11	11	22
variable		2	2
unknown		3	3
Paroxysmal abnormalities			
none	8	4	12
focal	6	7	13
multifocal	17	11	28
associated generalized	4	6	10
only generalized	0	0	0

Photosensitvity was progressively less apparent. Nevertheless it persisted in some cases and was observed in 12% of patients older than 18 years in one series (Bureau & Dalla Bernardina, 2011).

Neurological signs and motor ability

These aspects are not systematically described in the literature. Only ataxia was regularly reported and estimated to be present in more than one third of adults *(Table VII)*. Tremor and clumsiness of fine movements were also present in around one third of patients. Dysarthria was frequent in our patients. Pyramidal signs, including spasticity, Babinski sign, and enhanced deep tendon reflexes, were infrequent. Unexpectedly, some patients had extrapyramidal signs including rigidity, dystonic postures, and dystonic gait. In our series, interictal myoclonus persisted in eleven patients and disappeared in nine.We had no information for the remaining four.

In fact, often these patients have reduced motor abilities due to the combination of neurological signs and skeletal abnormalities which can lead to a peculiar posture developing into what was named "a crouch gait" by I. Scheffer (personal communication). Kyphosis and kypho-scoliosis, claw and, more often, flat feet contribute to walking difficulties, which were observed in seven patients in our series. Such difficulties were not obvious in childhood, became prominent during adolesence and worsened during subsequent years, in spite of physiotherapy. Two patients received surgery for kyphosis with a transitory benefit. Seven patients had severe walking impairment and two used a wheelchair. Akiyama *et al.* (2010) described two patients who were bedridden, at 43 and 31 years, respectively, without providing details about this very unusual outcome. It is interesting to underline that patients with the most severe motor handicap also have severe mental impairment.

Conversely, no motor disability was observed in four of the patients reported by Akiyama *et al.* (2010), three of those described by Jansen *et al.* (2006) and four in our series.

Results of neuroimaging are shown in *Table VIII.*

Table VII. *Neurological signs in adult patients.*

Study	Patients	Interictal myoclonia	Ataxia	Tremor-clumsiness	Dysarthria	Pyramidal signs.	Extra pyramid. signs
Jansen *et al.*, 2006	14	?	4	4	?	6	4
Dravet *et al.*, 2009	20 (a)	11	9	7	8	4	3
Akiyama *et al.*, 2010	31	?	13	11	?	?	?
Total	65	26	22				

(a) no information for four patients

Table VIII. *MRI findings at follow-up.*

	Akiyama *et al.*, 2010 29 pts		Jansen *et al.*, 2006 10 pts		Dravet *et al.*, 2009 15 pts		Total 54 pts	
MRI characteristics								
Normal	28		6		10		44	
Abnormal	1		4		3		8	
*diffuse brain atrophy		1		2		1		4
*localized atrophy						2		2
*hippocampal atrophy		0		2		0		2
Normal → abnormal					2		2	
*cerebellar atrophy						1		1
*subarachnoid spaces dilation						1		1

Cognitive, behavioural and social outcome

In most patients, there is no further cognitive decline after the first years of life but patients tend not to progress or progress slowly. Therefore, the gap between acquired and expected skills increases with age and cognitive level, as expressed by IQ scores, decreases. Thus, a child who appears to be slightly delayed at preschool age, could exhibit severe cognitive impairment in adolescence and adulthood. The motor disability described above tends to worsen with age, contributing to a decrease in adaptation for the needs of daily life. One characteristic feature is the extreme slowness in movement, verbal expression, comprehension and thinking. Language impairment is constant, but of variable degree. Sometimes, it is possible to have a conversation on simple topics concerning daily activities but the language remains poor and dysarthric, with verbal stereotypies and echolalia. Some patients are non-verbal and merely produce isolated syllables, words and inarticulate sounds or shouting. *Table IX* summarises the data reported by us and by Akiyama *et al.* (2010).

Table IX. *Language in adult patients.*

Dravet *et al.*, 2009	24 pts	Akiyama et al., 2010	31 pts
Relatively structured, communicative	7 pts	Simple conversation	5 pts
Not structured but communicative	7 pts	Primitive conversation	9 pts
		Able to speak several words	9 pts
Not communicative	4 pts		
No language	3 pts	No language	7 pts
?	3 pts	Minimal disability, psychotic	1 pt

Usually, these patients are rather calm and passive, searching affectionate contact with others and perseverating in repetitive activities. Nevertheless, in some, behavioural problems emerge such as obsessive attitudes, bouts of aggressiveness, nocturnal agitation, and, rarely, acute psychiatric episodes.

In a subset of patients, mental and behavioural aggravation occurs after adolescence. This was observed by Akiyama *et al.* (2010) in five patients; four with associated motor disorders and persistent severe epilepsy and one after disappearance of the seizures. We did not observe a similar pattern in our series of 24 patients. Although this situation sometimes occurs in our current practice, it is not definitive and these patients may improve again.

Gobbi *et al.* (2008) reported one episode of catatonic psychosis which occurred in a girl with preexisting autistic features. At 14 years, coinciding with a period of seizure-freedom after a change in her treatment, her behaviour quickly worsened. This episode subsided after reduction of AEDs and reappearance of some seizures. The authors attributed this episode to the "forced normalisation" of the EEG induced by treatment change.

These reduced abilities also affect *accomplishment in daily life activities*. In our series, only three patients were autonomous in daily life, eight were partially dependent, and 13 completely dependent. Consequently, only one woman could live in an "assisted living" apartment with support from a social worker. Eleven patients lived at home with their parents and attended either an occupational day centre, a sheltered workshop or a special "professional" school. Twelve patients were institutionalised in special centres for disabled people. Three did not have any social activity. In general, adult patients with DS did not have aggressive behaviour compromising their social integration, but their motor disability, difficulty to communicate, tendency to perseverate and refusal behaviour made them socially isolated.

In the Australian study (Jansen *et al.*, 2006), some patients were less severely impaired. One had low IQ scores, two had mild intellectual disability and two lived independently but were unemployed. One patient was engaged and one had a two-year-old daughter. However, the majority (10 patients) were not independent.

In the above studies, patients exhibited either typical DS or borderline forms. No significant differences in the long-term outcome emerged between these two groups. Genetic analysis was performed for most patients (54/69) and the majority carried a *SCN1A* gene mutation (40/54). Akiyama *et al.* did not find a relationship between seizure disappearance and any particular *SCN1A* mutation in five patients. However, a correlation between less severe intellectual disability and presence of occipital alpha rhythm on EEG was identified at follow-up. Intellectual disability was less severe in 4/5 seizure-free patients *vs* 11/26 patients with active epilepsy, although this difference was not statistically significant.

How to diagnose SMEI in adults

There are no absolute criteria for the diagnosis of SMEI in adults and not all patients present with the same characteristics. However, there are some features indicative of SMEI in adults with epilepsy.

Adult patients with DS present as disabled individuals, always slow in movement, language and thinking. They can walk, but often with difficulty and some must use a wheelchair for long distances. Their speech is slow and dysarthric and may sometimes lack sentence structure. Some patients have no language at all. Most adult patients exhibit mild to severe cognitive impairment, sometimes associated with psychotic traits. Motor impairment is almost constant, with a combination of ataxia, myoclonus, and clumsiness. Severe skeletal deformities can be present, such as kyphosis and kypho-scoliosis. Most patients are usually dependent on others and often live in specialised institutions.

Epilepsy is severe, with frequent nocturnal GTCS, often sensitive to fever. In some patients, atypical absences, myoclonic and focal seizures are occasionally observed. Seizures can be grouped in clusters for two or three days. Unlike LGS, sudden drop attacks are not usually seen but patients do fall to the ground when experiencing a GTCS during the day. Repetitive, purely axial tonic seizures during sleep are not observed. EEG does not show specific patterns. Background is normal or slow, and paroxysmal abnormalities are focal and multifocal. These patients have received heavy polytherapy treatments during their whole life. MRI is normal or shows slight cerebral or cerebellar atrophy, rarely hippocampal sclerosis. Confronted with such a patient, careful history taking provides recognition of SMEI and genetic analysis can be proposed.

Such a picture, which is indicative of a very unfavourable outcome, is observed in patients who were diagnosed a long time ago, often several years after epilepsy onset, and who did not receive an adequate teatment. We are aware of a small subset of patients who have experienced less severe disability, as also illustrated in an Autralian study by Jansen *et al.* (2006). As already mentioned, a good outcome was also reported by Buoni *et al.* (2006) in a young man. In our more recent patients, whose diagnosis was established earlier, more appropriate and efficacious drugs were used and a better seizure control was obtained, with reduction of seizure frequency and duration, particularly of episodes of status. These patients, who are still children or adolescents, also benefit from a more stimulating environment and rehabilitation and seem to be less delayed with less severe behavioural disorders. Although completely normal cognitive development remains exceptional, younger patients may achieve higher cognitive skills and a higher level of autonomy.

Mortality

DS is associated with a mortality rate amongst the highest in the epilepsy population and death may occur at any age, but more frequently during childhood. In studies which considered mortality in patients with epilepsy, the different epilepsy types were poorly defined and this rare type of childhood epilepsy was not individualised.

As a consequence, there are no informative epidemiological studies of mortality in DS and data in the literature are heterogeneous. Retrospective studies are also scarcely informative because of unavoidable biases. Only one prospective study would provide valuable results.

We have, however, tried to approach this topic which is a source of major worries for families and doctors. In 2005, we made a review of the literature published between 1982 and 2001.

We found 26 reported deaths and estimated the global mortality rate to be approximately 17.5% (Dravet *et al.*, 2005a, b). Causes of death were epileptic status in 11 patients (42.3% of all deaths), sudden unexpected death (SUDEP) in four (15.4%), and drowning, accident, infection, and unknown causes in the remaining patients.

In 2009, we conducted a survey including 36 centres in 13 countries. Among 903 patients, 52 had died (5.75%). The major cause was SUDEP, which had occurred in 28 (53.8% of all deaths). The remaining deaths included: epileptic status in six (25%), infection in five, drowning in four, complications of a seizure in three, accident in one, liver failure in one, and unknown in four. The mortality rate appeared to be lower in this population than in a smaller population between 1982 and 2001, with a higher proportion of SUDEP and a lower proportion of epileptic status.

A survey was conducted in Japan by Sakauchi *et al.* (2011). These authors sent a questionnaire to 246 children's hospitals and received 91 responses. Among the 623 patients followed at these centres, 63 deaths (10%) were reported. Data from 59 of these patients were analyzed. Death had been attributed to SUDEP in 53%, acute encephalopathy with epileptic status in 36%, drowning in 10% and fulminant hepatitis C in one patient.

An additional study was realised by the IDEA League which collected information on 833 individuals with DS, present in the IDEA League membership database in June 2010 (Skluzacek *et al.*, 2011). Among them, 31 were known to have died between 2000 and 2010 (3.72%); 19 by SUDEP (61.3% of all deaths), 10 by epileptic status (32.2%), one by a seizure-related accident, and one by keto-acidosis.

Results concerning SUDEP are remarkably similar in the three studies described above, with regards to incidence *(Table X)* and age of occurrence, mainly between two and ten years *(Figure 30)*. Differences concerning the other causes cannot really be estimated given the different methodologies. Using Kaplan-Meyer survival analysis, Skluzacek *et al.* (2011) found cumulative mortality rates by age 18 among children with DS in the IDEA League which were as follows: 2.9% SUDEP, 3.9% epileptic status, and 7.0% death by any cause. The annual incidence of SUDEP ranged from 0% to 1.3% with a mean annual rate of 0.6%, which is much higher than the average rates in children with unspecified epilepsy (Donner *et al.*, 2001; McGregor & Wheeless, 2006).

Table X. *Mortality synthesis.*

Origin	Patients (number)	Deaths (%)	SUDEP (%)	ES (%)	Others (%)
Sakauchi *et al.*, 2011	623	10	**53**	36	11
IDEA LEAGUE, 2010	833	3.72	**61.3**	32.2	6.4
Dravet *et al.*, 2005a, b	903	5.7	**53.8**	11.5	34.6

ES: epileptic status.

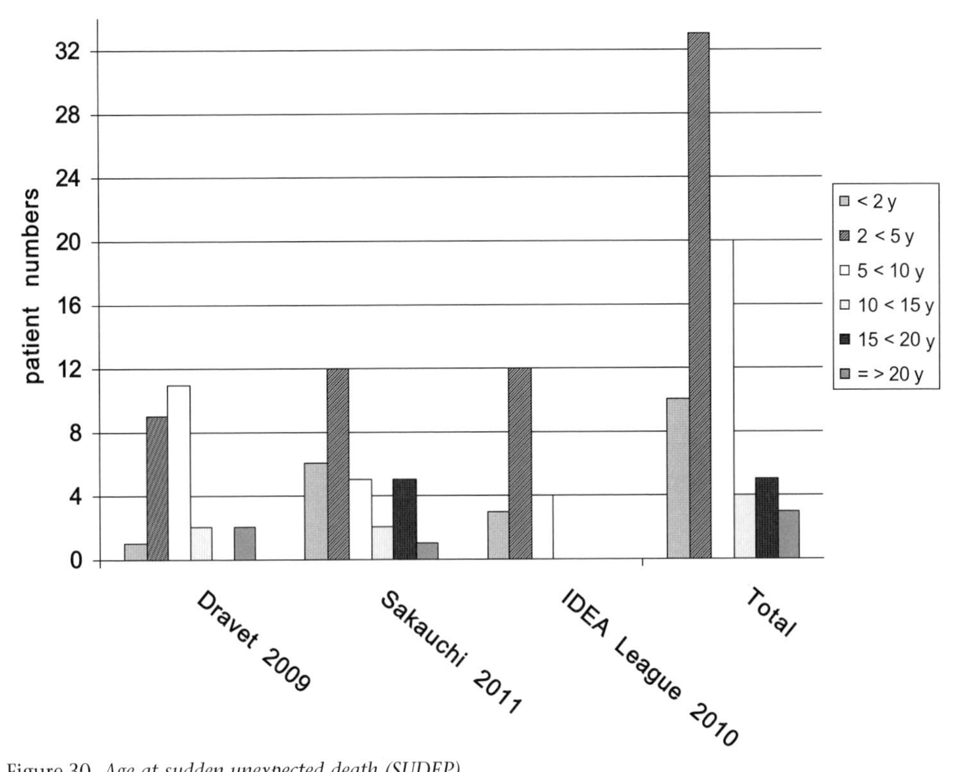

Figure 30. *Age at sudden unexpected death (SUDEP).*

The circumstances of SUDEP were those which were generally reported; most often, occurrence during sleep and in children who did not have recent aggravation and who received their treatment regularly, usually poytherapy. The numerous studies on this subject have failed to elucidate the mechanisms of SUDEP, although cardio-respiratory dysfunction has been hypothesized (Delogu *et al.*, 2011). Although preventative measures are not available, however, simple precautions can decrease the risk, such as frequent monitoring of the child when asleep, avoidance of the prone position, and the use of smoother pillows in order to try to minimise the consequences of respiratory obstruction and depression.

In the studies with adult patients, the rate of deaths was also high; 1/14 (Jansen *et al.*, 2006) and 5/24 (Dravet *et al.*, 2009). In the latter study, the cause of death was SUDEP in three patients, acute pneumopathy with epileptic status in one, and unknown in one. Six out 37 patients of Akiyama *et al.* (2010) had died between 5 and 12 year-old and the causes of death were SUDEP in one, pneumonia in two, and status epilepticus or seizure cluster in three.

Fortunately, this problem of mortality is now considered very seriously and numerous studies are being carried out to understand the mechanisms of SUDEP in epilepsy. Epileptic status is still frequent in DS, but by using more recent drugs, particularly stiripentol, and better management, the occurrence of status, as well as associated fatalities, should progressively decrease.

9. Case Reports and Words from Parents

Words from parents

In this chapter, we present examples of descriptions of DS that illustrate the true experiences of patients and families. We chose to let the parents themselves express their view of seizures, behaviour, results of treatment, management, and supporting groups.

The following quotations are taken from the forums where parents of children with DS communicate amongst each other. Only the children's names have been removed, and we have just made a few typographical corrections. These quotations show how the parents accurately observe their children's seizures and behaviour, and they desire to share their experience and observations with other parents in order to break their isolation and better understand their children and the disease.

Seizures

Atypical absence seizure

D. 14 months

* His myoclonics seem to be not as noticeable as before, but he still has them. They seem to be limited to the eyebrows now. It is hard to explain, but I am starting to think that it could be absences, not sure. They are very short, about one second. He has jerking of the eyebrows and a blank stare for a second. It is so short that I still can't understand what it is exactly. He also does the same thing during his seizures, his eyebrows jerk with a blank stare, in exactly the same way.

Obtundation status

* He can also have a type of seizure that gives him a cloudy look with very slight body jerks from side to side (not up and down), lasting about two to three seconds. Interestingly, recently, he had a weird seizure that started in exactly the same way; he was standing up, jerking from side to side, with cloudy eyes. After a couple of minutes of jerking, his consciousness was kind of impaired and he looked "silly" and in 20 minutes he became completely unresponsive.

Falsely generalised convulsive seizure

* More often, he has seizures that I think Dr Dravet calls falsely generalised, but I am not sure...

It starts with facial jerking just seconds before he becomes stiff, but not like in "true" tonic phase, it looks weird. He straightens his hands forward and a bit down, and his body looks as if it is folded for a couple of seconds. His mouth is open; that really amazes me, because it is supposed to be shut in tonic phase, then clonic phase starts. His eyes are always open, sometimes turned to the side, sometimes looking straight forward. He loses consciousness gradually. So it is obviously not a true tonic-clonic. I also think it could be, sort of, partial seizures that look like generalised seizures, but I don't really know. Doctors have always said it was grand mal, because they only see the last part.

Complex partial seizure

* My daughter is now six and a half years old. Today, she just came home from a three-day video EEG. The neuro arranged one for her as we have been seeing a lot of aura or complex partial seizure-like episodes for over a year. She becomes very confused and looks scary with her face becoming flushed. On many occasions, she can still respond "OK" when we ask her. She can even follow our instructions to close her eyes and take a deep breath. From the VEEG results, which indicated four seizures from the last three days, they are all focal and complex partial seizures, from 10 seconds to three minutes.

Postictal behaviour

* My son (almost four) has also experienced large achievements after prolonged seizures. His tonic-clonics always go into status, but we are usually able to stop them with Diastat [Diazepam rectal gel for the treatment of breakthrough seizures at home – Authors' note]. I have noticed, a week or so before he has a tonic-clonic, that his behaviour is more erratic (shorter attention spans, misbehaving, *etc.*) and he becomes clumsier. It almost seems like the seizure "reboots" his brain- I wonder if there is just so much static and chaos going on in their brains prior to the seizure that it becomes hard to concentrate....

When he was sick this last time, he went almost a whole day without speaking which I attributed to a sore throat. In the early evening, he had a tonic-clonic and we administered diastat. When he awoke, he went back to chatting as normal. I think perhaps all the latent seizure activity just makes it hard on them and the seizure is almost like a release on a pressure valve that sets things back to normal.

Triggering factors

* Welcome to the group. My son is 14 years old and we have been through *a lot of different things* over the years; of different things that would trigger seizures for him. You have already noted that temperature is a big thing for a child with Dravet. A lot of kids will have seizures in water if the temperature of the water is too hot or too cold. Some kids cannot even have a bath without having a seizure. As for the car, it could be sunlight flickering through the trees. We found that T. was extremely photosensitive and pattern sensitive when he was younger. Rather than going into a whole lot of information right now, I would think about having your son wear sunglasses outside and in the car, if you can get him to wear a broad brimmed hat it might be useful.

Light

* Our experience with M. is similar. When he was younger we had to be careful if we were driving in areas where there were trees, as the sunlight through the trees would create this dappled effect that would irritate him. Polarised glasses would be helpful for her if this is the cause.

* L. is very photosensitive, but on a 20-minute EEG when lights were flashed at her, she showed no sensitivity. Other times, I've had to ask them to stop because she was so distressed. Apparently photosensitivity can come and go.

Emotion, stress

* My daughter has for a long time, suffered from atypical absences (eyelid fluttering) and myoclonic jerks. Mostly, these are brought on by stress, but only a tiny amount is necessary. For instance, at a party this week, about 15 minutes from the end, she started to jerk and flutter, obviously wanting to go home. We waited until the end, but once out of the door, she skipped to the car and was perfectly fine for the rest of the day. Yesterday, we went out for the day, after playing happily for an hour, we went indoors to eat and she wanted to go on a bouncy castle. She started taking her shoes off, I told her no, we were going to have dinner and she started jerking and fluttering, climbed onto my knee and eventually went to sleep. We have about two or three incidences like this a week. She doesn't cry, scream or shout or lose her temper, she jerks.

Water, temperature

* With the pool, it is the getting in and getting out with a drastic temperature change (only a couple degree differences between the two) that we have to be most concerned about. He could not get too hot or too cold. We usually have someone on standby to throw a towel around him immediately and that helps prevent a seizure. I will say for him, both of these triggers have improved with age.

* My daughter with Dravet is 13. We LOVE the beach and vacation there every summer. It was really hard when F. was young. She was unable to tolerate the cold water or the bright sun. When we were at the beach I would let her step her toes in the surf and then we hung out under the umbrella in the sand. She couldn't be out in the hot part of the day and always had sunglasses on. By the grace of God, the sun is NO LONGER an issue- it's truly a miracle! F. can swim on the sunniest of days now. She doesn't wear sunglasses either! Temperature of the water is still an issue but not to the same extent. Now she can tell me when it is too cold, and we don't go in.

Physical exercise, temperature

* Sorry for butting in but we also have a huge problem with L. my 4-year-old. If she plays, runs, jumps, anything like that for longer than 10 minutes she will have a seizure... How do you tell a child to calm down, this is one of our most difficult issues.

* Anything that requires any level of exertion triggers seizures for W. Trampoline, swinging on bars, running, dancing, climbing, gymnastics, kicking a ball... and more I'm sure.

* My daughter, now 10 years old, still has seizures related to water temp. and body temp.

* Anything that makes her temperature go above 37 is a trigger.

* She does have a cooling vest she wears when she goes outside because she doesn't sweat and so overheats very quickly. You can find them at www.coolsport.net.

Neurological and motor signs

* I am thinking that A's walking and posture is a natural progression of Dravet: knees turning in, upper body leaning forward from hips. T. wears orthotics in his shoes, but nothing else. Although not mentioned in studies, T. is also tending to have his head down a lot of the time, to the point where it needs to be physically held up so that I can listen to what he is saying or put meds in his mouth.

* I am the mother of a 4-year-old daughter named H. We are also noticing this with her. H. has always walked a little funny [...]. Recently her knees have started to turn in and when she is really tired she leans forward from the hips up, she walks very flat-footed and has started dragging her feet more. For me, being around her 24/7 makes it harder to notice this stuff because I am always looking at her, so the progression is slow.

* P. is 10 and a half years old. He is still having gait issues, but we have decided to give him a break on orthotics over the summer. The last orthopaedic doc said that even when we use them regularly, there is only so much they can do, as for a typical child the muscles are more like rubber bands, whereas for our kids they are like bungee cords. Since they are so lax, there is not much that can be done to address the splaying. He is not displaying a crouch gait yet, but definitely that weird Dravet gait that I know a lot of us are familiar with. We have been advised to work on shoulder and trunk strength as he has started to walk with curved shoulders.

Learning, behaviour

* Just thinking about what you were saying here, about our kids being obsessed with certain tasks and doing things over and over again. J. does the same, he has favourite toys and jigsaws that he will do over and over for an hour and sometimes more. Especially if he is getting a reaction and some sort of praise. I tended to think of it as autistic tendencies associated with his lack of development (disability), not the SMEI.

* We get full mobility allowance for J. He can walk but due to his behaviour and seizures we take him everywhere in his major buggy... J. is quite mobile, he can climb and run although he looks like he is going to wobble over and crash at any minute... He used to want to walk but would have a seizure walking anywhere further than about 150 metres; so I used to let him walk the last bit of the way on the way home but he always had one of those children straps on. I used to be petrified he would seize on me, and a lot of the time he did, but he was adamant that he wanted to walk.

* LOL, new name for SMEI – Little Monkeys that Climb Syndrome (LMCS)! N. is like Tarzan with a bit of Houdini added in! We are having the stairs blocked in – because she uses the spindles as a climbing frame and no matter how many times she falls or I say "no", she still carries on! We have a huge piece of perspex covering her bedroom window at the moment for the same reason, just until her room is finished.

* C. is now six and a half years old. Major concern is still her autistic features and she is very weak in spontaneous conversation and play skills. Very often, she can be socially odd, especially at her current age. Though she can speak in complete sentences, she displays a very stereotyped communication. Yet she is still a very cheerful and easy-to-manage person.

* Just watched some home videos of my son when he was two. He was so alert, talkative, bright, and engaged. Now he is autistic, has language difficulties and is usually unengaged. It got me wondering, since he had the same genes then as he has now... what exactly causes the mental decline? And autism, why do some Dravet kids develop it and some don't.

I know this is part of the progression of the disease, but why? Are there any strong theories about exactly what causes this and why some kids are so much more affected than others?

* Ten and a half years old... His behaviour has got better. He tried and failed two behaviour meds, but then behaviour started to improve while he was not taking anything for it. I think it is partly because of the school and their work with his behaviour, but I also tend to believe that when he is at his worst behaviourally that perhaps there is some subclinical seizure activity going on. He will be doing something he knows he shouldn't and you can tell that he can't turn it off (if that makes sense).

Course and outcome

* E. had a bad first year of life, with some long seizures which were very hard to control, she then had a very good second year with nine months without a seizure, a really normal third year with one or two seizures, every three months only triggered with fever, but her fourth year was awful, the worst to date: a seizure every week, short- but we never knew what triggered them. Through that year we tried hundreds of meds, and doses, and finally E. is having a really good fifth year (touch wood).

* J. turned seven last month. He is still a lovely and very happy little boy. He is still on no medication (that's been three years now apart from the odd dose of clobazam as a semi-emergency med). He has about eight seizures a month, tonic-clonic, about two minutes long, in his sleep. His speech has still not returned although we keep thinking it's about to happen, he is not toilet trained and operates on about an 18 level, possibly more now.

* T. will be nine years old in August and is doing quite well. Most of her seizures are during sleep and few last more than 90 seconds. We usually get a week to 10 days a month break when she has none... It's been four years now since we've had to move her into our bed.

She is currently on stiripentol, valproic acid and clonazepam, along with monthly IVIG treatments. It's been the IVIG that seems to have given us this current stability.

Because of the reduced seizure activity, T. is learning well. She's in Grade 3 but has a fully modified program. Her reading and maths skills are at a mid-grade 1 level. I constantly remind the teachers and school staff that our first priority is socialisation... Her social age now is about four and a half. She loves to play with baby dolls, play piano and lots of games!

* D. is approaching her teenage years (she will be 13 in November). Regardless, she is still so vulnerable, and almost too trusting of people... which is often one of my worries. She too, never had any fear as a young kid, and still is not quite aware of the real consequences of some things. She is almost too trusting of people.

* B. is 14, turning 15 in August. She'll be going into Grade 10 (high school) in September. We've hit our plateau at an average of one big seizure a night. Over a week, she will typically have 1, 3, 2, 1, 1, 0, 0 seizures in a night. I haven't been able to figure out any triggers that

set it off. She has such variable days and sleep times that I can't see what sets off the pattern of seizures.

But right now, she's happy, loves piling things, and likes playing with jigsaw puzzles. She has lost her addiction to completing the puzzles. She is now more interested in taking the pieces out of the boxes and putting them back in (or throwing them one by one across the room). Same thing with her bucket of crayons.

Her walking is fairly predictable. And when she's doing really well, she has a sort of skipping gait that she enjoys (and gives me heart attacks). She is currently on stiripentol, topiramate and clonazepam, with warfarin at night. And things are good.

* H. is in grade 6 now – and she is able to interact with her classmates very well. She plays with a few of the children in her class (intermittently) but also plays with the younger children – who she loves to dote over. Her classmates are accepting and caring – but they don't always go out of their way to play with her... Her age level (mindset) is a few years younger and so she doesn't share a lot of similarities with some of the kids. She is very outspoken... You wouldn't know it really – that C. was any different – until you've talked to her for a bit... She can memorise very well. With practice, she can actually stand up there on stage, or in front of the class – and make a presentation, or recite a poem or prayer (just like any other her age... and sometimes even better).

* A. is now 14 and a half years old and for about five years has been doing relatively well. I am posting this to give some hope to other families as we too have been through some very tough times... She is actually on less medicine than when she was three years old and she weighs 100 lbs more. I give her a lot of supplements, including magnesium (which I firmly believe is just as important as her meds), B6, calcium+D, multivit and fish oil. A. wants to be a teacher's assistant one day, or at least work in preschool. She loves ice skating and once she learns front crossovers and can spin more than one rotation, I will look into special Olympics. She is social, and loves to be with friends. She will be going into a LifeSkills class next year for high school and she is looking forward to working in the school store and going into the community. She does have many typical teen moments, and gets irritated easily, and is immature. Her language is not always that clear, but she gets her point across. She can read at a 2nd-3rd grade level and her maths is perhaps slightly lower. Just to let you know that A. still has two to three blinkies a day (eye fluttering seizures) but we ignore them. Her last big seizures were last summer when both meds switched to generic the same week. These seizures were only four minutes and stopped on their own – considering we were used to one to three hours of status absence and 20-minute partial complex seizures, this was not too bad. She also has a VNS in which the battery died in the past year with no significant worsening so we haven't replaced the battery... I am always hoping and praying that as all our children age, the seizures will become more manageable and then we can all enjoy our children for who they are and not have to worry quite so much.

Support groups

* J. turned seven last month. He is still a lovely and very happy little boy. I continue to meet up with lots of Dravet families. It is always so amazing how much the children have in common – and the parents too. I would never have wished to meet any one of you and not

to have lived with Dravet but, seeing as we don't have any choice in that, it is wonderful to be part of this one big family.

* She has made a lot of advance in her development this summer. She rides her bike now, very strong and fast, and it has been the greatest gift God has given me this year. Seeing her riding her bike in the street, with her brother is great. I share this with you, because I never thought she would be able to ride a bike, and she is... just for those who are not so well now... don't lose the hope.

* Since taking him off lamictal, I am happy to tell you all that he has been seizure-free since March 12 – the longest he has ever gone without seizures is three weeks when he started clobazam about a year ago, so to be heading into two and a half months of seizure freedom is a miracle... I write this to those of you whose children are on lamictal – not that you take them off, as I know some who are doing quite well, but just as a FYI and reference. Each of our precious children is different and what works for one is not going to work for another but I just wanted you to know my experience.

Case reports

First patient

F. was born on November 15th, 1985, from healthy parents. He was brought to our attention at the age of four and a half and is now 26 years old.

There is no family history of epilepsy or febrile seizures. His younger sister is healthy.

He presented his first episode at seven months, during moderate hyperthermia. It was a generalised tonic-clonic seizure (GTCS) lasting 10 minutes, followed by a second episode five minutes apart. In spite of VPA treatment, seizures recurred every 2-3 months during the first three years of life. These were either generalised or lateralised, alternatively left and right, and lasted up to 20 minutes. Atypical absences appeared at around the third year of life but disappeared at age four after steroid treatment, whereas GTCS persisted, mainly during sleep. However, absences relapsed during childhood and frequent obtundation statuses occurred, often culminating in a GTCS. This patient never presented true myoclonic seizures but interictal multifocal myoclonic jerks were always observed, increasing just before a GTCS. The initial EEG recordings were normal. From age three years on, EEG showed numerous discharges of generalised spikes and waves (SW), and polyspikes and waves (PSW), later on associated with multifocal abnormalities and slow background activity. Several recorded seizures showed focal onset. Photic stimulation was ineffective. Seizures remained frequent, sometimes occurring in daily clusters till adulthood, in spite of various AED combinations. Only CLB appeared to reduce the myoclonic jerks for several years. At the age of 25 years, seizure frequency increased, leading to GTC status, which was interrupted by intravenous barbiturates.

Several brain MRI scans were normal.

Mutation analysis of the *SCN1A* gene revealed a heterozygous nucleotide deletion c.1846delG causing early interruption of the protein at amino acid 622 (E616delX622).

F. had normal early development. At three years of age, he spoke properly but exhibited peculiar behavioural traits. He acquired reading and writing skills but his abilities deteriorated in the following years, leaving him at an elementary level. He never acquired autonomy in daily life. At 26 years of age, his behaviour is now characterised by delayed thinking and speaking, language stereotypies, perseveration, and poor interest for his surroundings. Formal neuropsychological evaluation is impracticable. He lives with his parents, walks with "crouching" attitude, and has never had bouts of aggressiveness.

Conclusion. This patient is an example of the severe form of Dravet syndrome which has evolved as such in spite of normal development in early childhood.

Second patient

A. was born on July 20th, 1995, from healthy parents. She was followed up in our hospital for two years since she was 11 years old.

There was no family history of epilepsy or febrile seizures. Her older sister was healthy.

She presented her first seizure at age five months, appearing without fever after vaccine. This was a focal motor clonic attack of the left upper limb that lasted 15 minutes and was followed by transient left hemiparesis. Ten days later, she manifested a second focal seizure, involving the right upper limb, with secondary generalisation. EEG and CT scan revealed no abnormalities. After three more seizures occurring in the following days, she was put on carbamazepine (CBZ). Generalised clonic seizures persisted with a frequency of three per month, usually lasting for no longer than five minutes. From age 10 months on, brief myoclonic seizures with absences appeared. The EEG showed interictal bilateral fronto-central spikes and generalised SW, whereas brief discharges of generalised PSW were associated with the absences, usually triggered by photic stimulation. A diagnosis of Dravet syndrome was considered and CBZ was substituted by phenobarbital (PB) and valproate (VPA). In the following years, convulsive seizures decreased, appearing only during fever. However, myoclonic and absence seizures remained frequent, up to 400 per day, associated with complex focal seizures, and photosensitivity persisted. Various AEDs were ineffective (ETS, CLB, LTG, TPM, and ZNS), with the exception of VPA and LEV which appeared to control absences and myoclonic seizures for about two years.

At nine years of age, the girl presented again atypical absences and myoclonic jerks, triggered by looking at contrasting surfaces. These seizures became particularly disabling as such contrasting surfaces were ubiquitous (in the form of lines, squares, grills, and objects such as escalators and lifts, and knitted clothes). Combined VPA, LEV, TPM, and intermittent CLB were effective but due to side -effects TPM was suspended at 11 years of age. Several EEGs were performed, still showing the generalised and focal abnormalities, as well as photosensitivity that had previously been observed. Wearing the Z1 glasses inhibited the photoparoxysmal response during the EEG but controlled pattern sensitivity in everyday life only partially. Two brain MRI scans were normal.

Mutation analysis of the *SCN1A* gene revealed a. 4385A>G mutation c determining the amino acidic substitution p.Y1462C.

Developmental skills were said to be normal up to the age of three years, when the global developmental quotient (TDQ) was 105, the verbal quotient (VDQ) 112, and the performance quotient (PDQ) 125 (Griffiths Scale). Between age three and five years, stagnation was observed. At five years of age, visuo-motor integration, visuo-coordination and verbal skills were impaired (TDQ = 76). In the following years, the girl slowly progressed, but her IQ scores decreased to GIQ = 55, VIQ = 54, PIQ = 64 (WISC-R). She had attention, visuo-spatial and sequential thinking difficulties. However, she could elaborate her experience of epilepsy and benefited from psychotherapy. She has attended normal school with support from an individual teacher. She acquired reading and writing, but not mathematic skills. She has benefited from musicotherapy and several stimulating activities. She had normal relationships with her classmates and did not suffer from behavioural problems.

Conclusion. This is an example of a moderately severe syndrome, in which episodes of status epilepticus have not occurred. This is a factor that might explain the good development in the first years, before the appearance of myoclonic and absence seizures. However, pattern sensitivity and outcome at adolescence were typical.

THIRD PATIENT

G. was born in 2005, from healthy parents. She was first seen in our hospital at two years of age and is now five years and eight months old.

There is no family history of epilepsy or febrile seizures.

She presented her first seizure at five months, three hours after the second hexavalent vaccination. It was a focal seizure, with right upper limb clonic jerks and secondary generalisation, lasting 15 minutes. A post-ictal EEG showed abnormalities on the right hemisphere. Two weeks later, a second seizure occurred during an ear infection involving the left side, before generalisation. At age 9 months, after three more seizures, treatment with VPA was prescribed, but febrile and afebrile clonic seizures persisted. Their frequency was variable, from one to eight per month, often in clusters, always very brief (one to three minutes). She never had episodes of status epilepticus but did have sporadic atypical absences. Myoclonic jerks were sporadically recorded, associated with spike and wave discharges, during a EEG polygraphy. EEG while awake showed posterior alpha activity without abnormalities. There was no response to photic stimulation. VPA monotherapy was maintained and associated for one year with add on CLB.

Brain MRI scan was normal.

Molecular analysis revealed a c.5531delCAAA mutation of the SCN1A gene.

The girls' development was normal from the onset of the disorder and was still normal at five years and eight months of age. Different assessments provided the following results: TDQ = 125 at the age of three years, 126 at the age of four (Griffiths Scale), and TIQ = 115 at the age of five years (WWPPSI). At the last test, a significant difference appeared between verbal (121) and performance (96) IQ. She always had difficulties in hand-eye coordination and visual attention and benefited from psychomotor treatment. She also has some motor impairment and often walks on tiptoes. Conversely, language and social interaction are completely normal. Her behaviour is also appropriate for age.

Conclusion. This case provides an example of a non severe course of the syndrome, belonging to the borderline forms, without myoclonic seizures and without status epilepticus. Although clonic seizures were frequent, they were very short and the child did not received heavy AED treatments. The normal background EEG activity may be considered a favourable prognostic element.

Annexes

Annex 1: Extracts from evaluations of a ten-year-old boy

Speech therapy report

During the class, D. is hyperkinetic (locomotiv) and disruptive with limited periods of concentration. He has a tendency to stand up from the chair and explore the space around him, although an already familiar environment. He needs constant delimitation because otherwise he becomes manipulative and takes over. He often talks without pausing, and this talkativeness relates to both fairytales, that he knows by heart, and daily events. Sometimes he becomes aggressive by pulling the hair of others or by hitting their faces. He shows a strong attachment with the activities that he is familiar with and it is hard to utilise something new. He is rigid at every level of communication, verbal and non verbal.

Expressive speech. D. has developed expressive speech that lacks organisation of structure and length, and factual content. His speech is stereotyped and he cannot use it in a functional way, despite the fact that he is fully trained at the cognitive level. He does not open a dialogue and does not transfer information from his everyday life. Even when he starts a dialogue he doesn't stay on the subject and does not interact normally. He does not have a direct, verbal response. He has a rich passive and active lexical background which he does not take advantage of for his verbal communication. He understands simple concepts and has a difficulty understanding more complex ones.

Articulation. As far as his articulation is concerned, D. cannot pronounce the letters X, PS in addition to a number of symphonic complexes. A difficulty can also be observed in acoustically discriminating the letters F, TH, V, D (delta), T, and K. There is incomplete tongue mobility (only extrusion of the tongue on the outside) and salivation.

Comprehension. The level of D.'s comprehension cannot be fully measured due to his strong disruption. Nevertheless, he does follow simple commands and even more complex ones when he chooses to do so.

Concentration of attention. There is a considerable amount of difficulty in relation to concentration; at such a level that D. cannot use his acquired knowledge. Due to his strong disruption, his verbal memory is particularly problematic.

Learning abilities. D. has not acquired the mechanisms of writing and reading.

Physiotherapy report

D. moves quite freely. He walks with his head forward and his chin slightly projecting, his body slightly bent and his knees are also in a bent position. There is external rotation in his hip and valgus talipes in his feet, which is bigger on the left foot.

When he is standing up, his head is forward with his chin slightly projecting and he immobilizes his body with his pelvis tilted forward and his knees in an extended position.

He can go up and down stairs by holding on to the railing and walks quite normally.

He can manage to stay in a kneeling position and half-knee position without help. To stand up from the kneeling and half-knee position, he needs support.... From the standing position to the sitting position, he also needs support. He can stand on one foot but the balance reactions are lacking...

In the kneeling position he tilts his pelvis forward with his legs apart, but if he is asked he can correct this position. In this position he can play ball by throwing it without losing his balance...

Muscular tone of the body is hypotonic. In the supine position, normal flexions the head is lacking. Protective reactions of the upper limbs are also lacking due to slow reaction. He has normal range of passive movements to upper and lower limbs. There is increased muscular tone of the Achilles tendons. He uses sole pads to lessen the problem with the flat feet.

In spite of the problem of concentration, he manages to follow his physiotherapy exercises satisfactorily. He has been having physiotherapy for three years.

Annex 2: Drawings from patients

Examples of drawings performed, either spontaneously or on demand, by patients during the consultations.

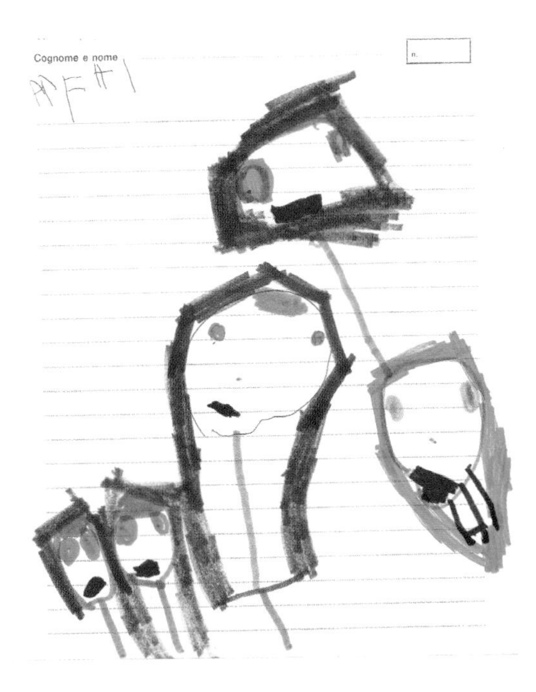

Figure 31. *Five-year, seven-month-old girl drew a picture of her family. She represented her mother in the middle, her father on the top, her two sisters on one side, and herself on the other side. Her image is very different from those of the others.*

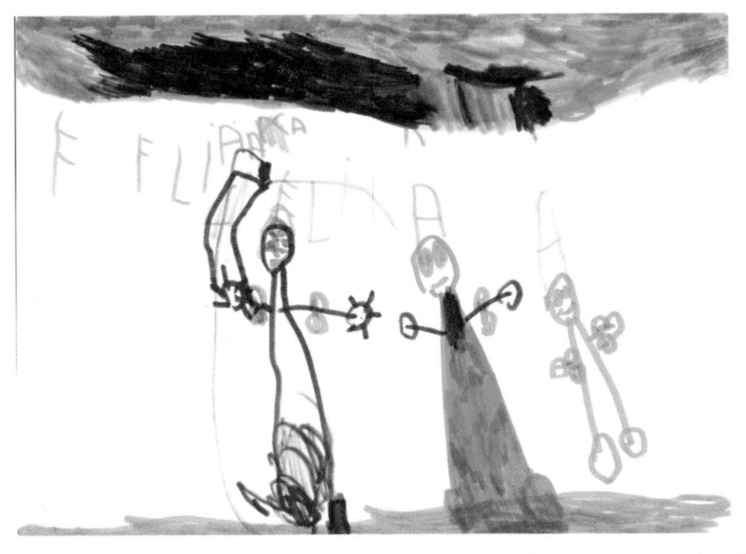

Figure 32. *The same girl when aged six years and six months. She drew three personages and tried to write her name. She made considerable progresses in one year.*

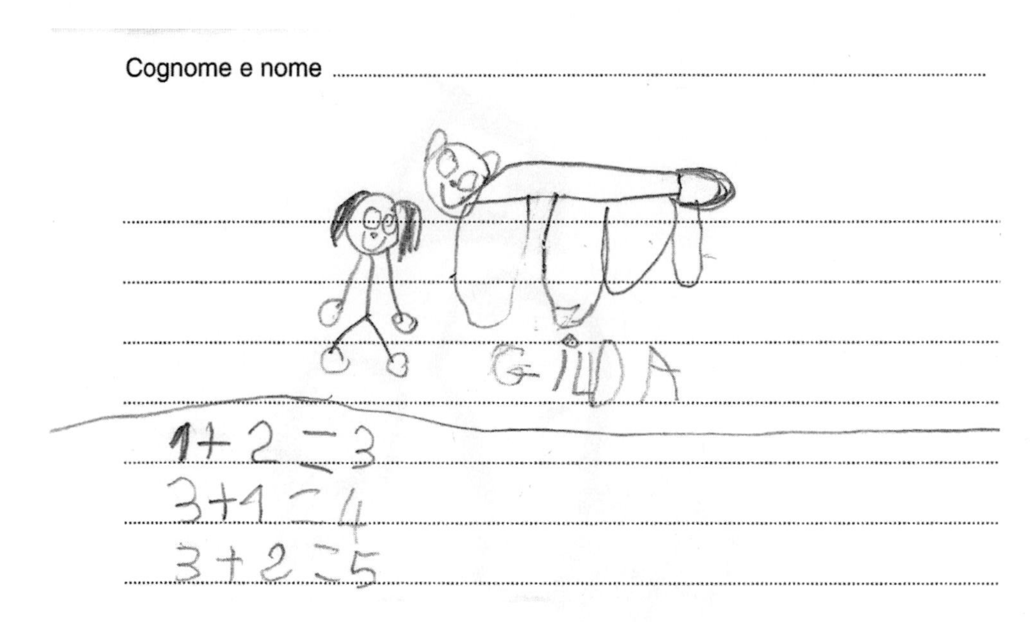

Figure 33. *Nine-year-old girl. Her representation of a dog and a child is schematic with surprising proportions. She was able to perform simple additions.*

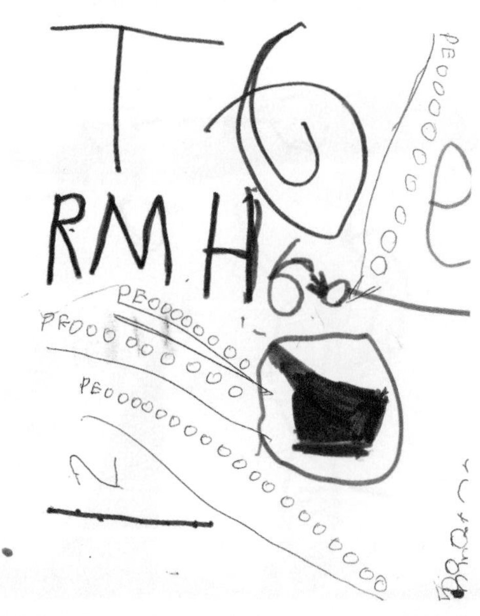

Figure 34. *Nine-year-old girl. Spontaneous writing, without meaning, as also recognized by the girl herself. She was able to speak but exhibited psychotic symptoms.*

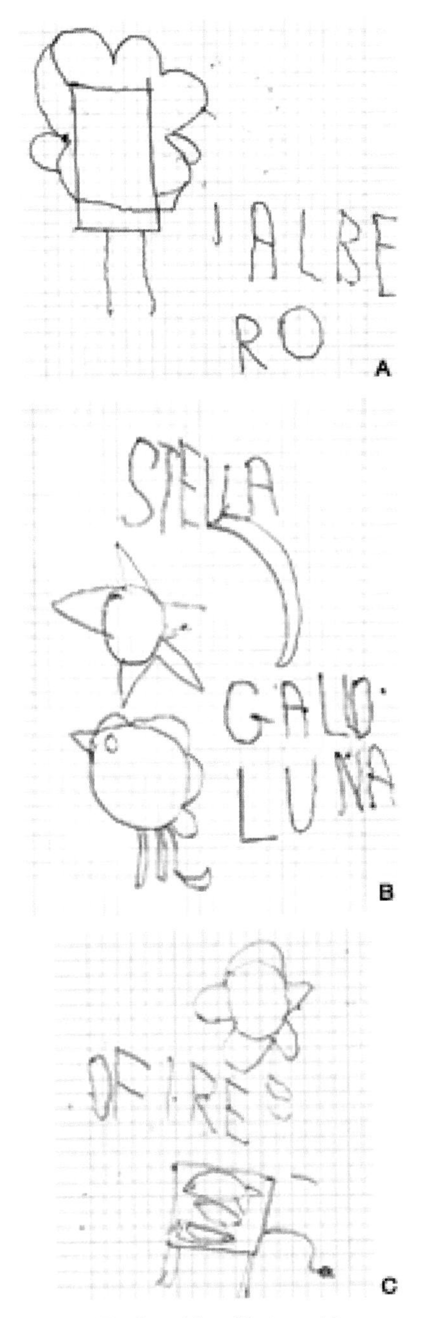

Figure 35a, b and c. *25-year-old man. He chose his subjects on his own and correctly described them. The drawings are of poor quality; the lines are irregular due to tremor.*

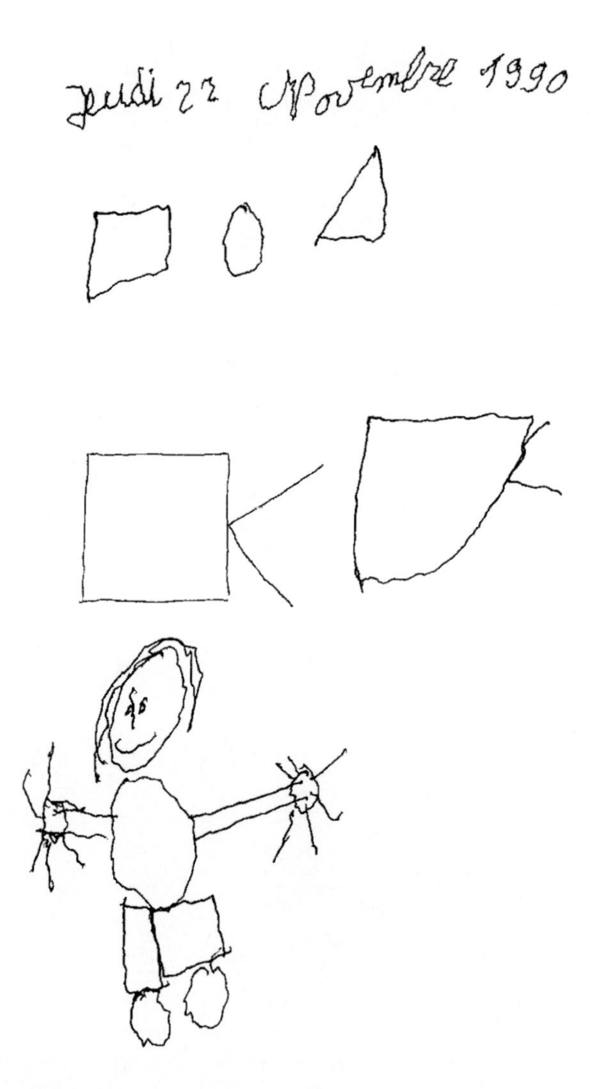

Figures 36 and 37. *Drawing realised by adolescents. Figure 36: 17-year-old man correctly writing the date, drawing three geometric figures, reproducing two others and drawing a personage.*

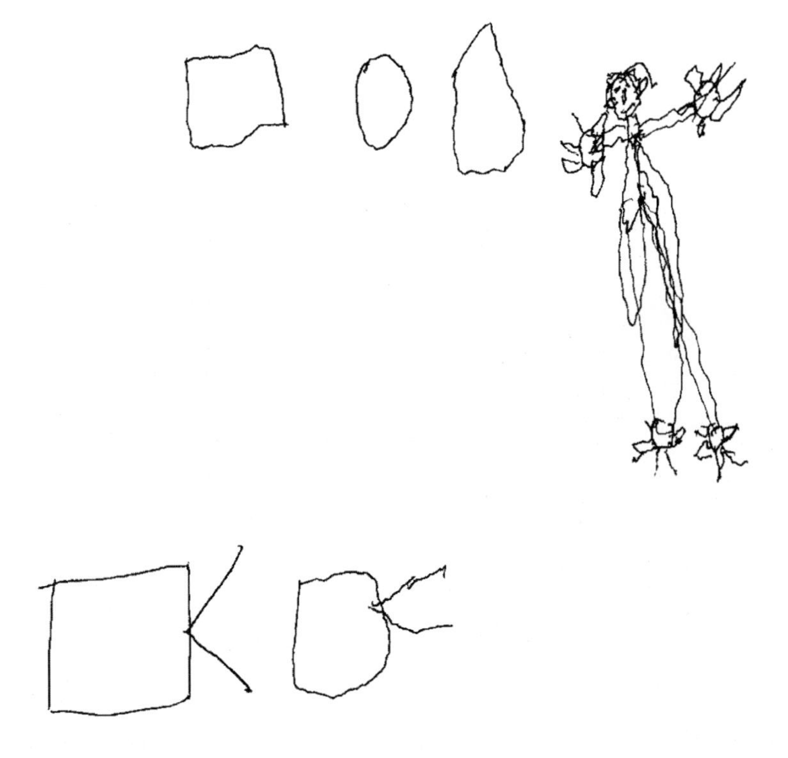

Figure 37: 15-year-old girl, drawing geometric figures and one personage. The two examples show visuo-perceptive and motor impairment with shaky lines, less marked in the girl.

ANNEX 3: SPECIAL GLASSES FOR PHOTOSENSITIVITY

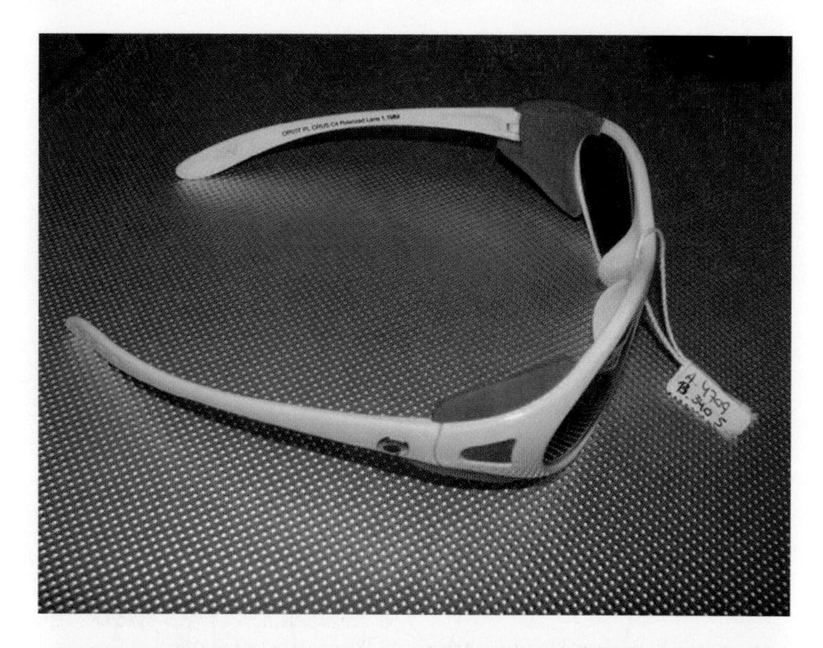

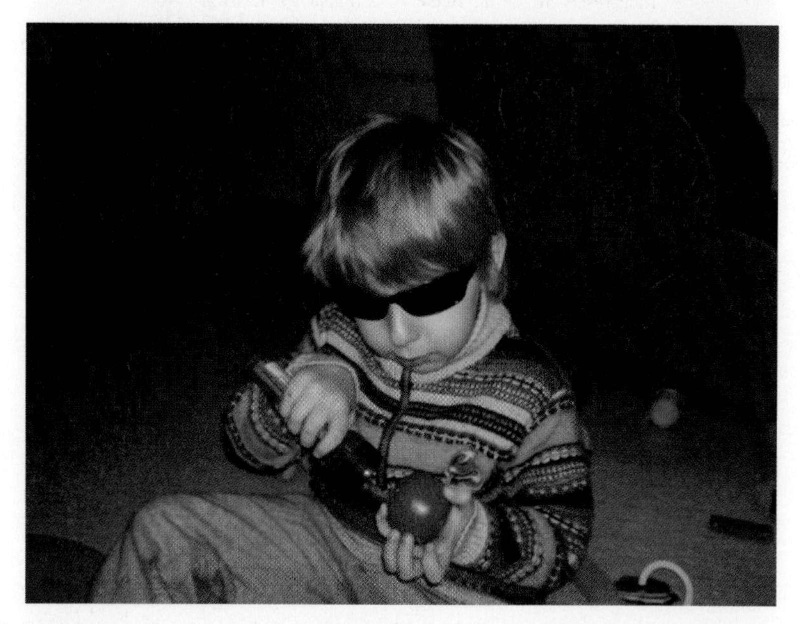

Figure 38. *Special glasses for photosensitive patients (reference Clarlet F133).*

References

• Abend NS, Gutierrez-Colina AM, Dlugos DJ. Medical treatment of pediatric status epilepicus. *Semin Pediatr Neurol* 2010; 17: 169-75.

• Aicardi J, Levi Gomes A. The myoclonic epilepsies of childhood. *Clev Clin J Med* 1989: S34-S39.

• Aicardi J. *Epilepsy in children (2nd edition).* New-York: Raven Press, 1994.

• Akiyama M, Kobayashi K, Yoshinaga H, Ohtsuka Y. A long-term follow-up study of Dravet syndrome up to adulthood. *Epilepsia* 2010; 51: 1043-52.

• Amin R, Ford-Jones E, Richardson SE, *et al.* Acute childhood encephalitis and encephalopathy associated with influenza. A prospective 11-year review. *Pediatr Infect Dis J* 2008; 27: 390-5.

• Andrade DM, Hamani C, Lozano AM, Wennberg RA. Dravet syndrome and deep brain stimulation: Seizure control after 10 years of treatment. *Epilepsia* 2010; 51: 1314-6.

• Awaya Y, Satoh F, Miyamoto M, Kayashii K, Inaba R, Fukuyama Y. Change of rectal temperature in infants and children during and after hot water immersion. *Clinical Thermometry* (Tokyo) 1989; 9: 76-82.

• Benloumis A, Nabbout R, Feingold J, *et al.* Genetic predisposition to severe myoclonic epilepsy in infancy. *Epilepsia* 2001; 42: 204-9.

• Berg AT, Berkovic SF, Brodie MJ, *et al.* Revised terminology and concepts of the organization of seizures and epilepsies: Report of the ILAE commission on classification and terminology, 2005-2009. *Epilepsia* 2010; 51: 676-85.

• Berkovic SF, Harkin L, McMahon JM, *et al. De-novo* mutations of the sodium channel gene *SCN1A* in alleged vaccine encephalopathy: A retrospective study. *Lancet Neurol* 2006; 5: 488-92.

• Buoni S, Orrico A, Galli L, *et al. SCN1A* (2528delG) novel truncating mutation with benign outcome of severe myoclonic epilepsy of infancy. *Neurology* 2006; 66: 606.

• Bureau M, Dalla Bernardina B. Electroencephalographic characteristics of Dravet Syndrome. *Epilepsia* 2011; 52 (Suppl. 2): 13-23.

• Capovilla G, Gambardella A, Rubboli G, *et al.* Suppressive efficacy by a commercially available blue lens on PPR in 610 photosensitive epilepsy patients. *Epilepsia* 2006; 47: 529-33.

• Caraballo R, Cersosimo R, Galicchio S, Fejerman N. Epilepsias en el primer año de vida. *Rev Neurol* (Barcelone) 1997; 25: 1521-4.

• Caraballo RH, Fejerman N. Dravet syndrome: A study of 53 patients. *Epilepsy Res* 2006; 70 (Suppl. 1): S231-8.

• Caraballo RH. Nonpharmacologic treatments of Dravet syndrome: Focus on the ketogenic diet. *Epilepsia* 2011; 52 (Suppl. 2): 79-82.

• Cassé-Perrot C, Wolff M, Dravet C. Neuropsychological aspects of severe myoclonic epilepsy in infancy. In: Jambaqué I, Lassonde M, Dulac O (eds). *The Neuropsychology of Childhood Epilepsy.* New-York: Plenum Press/Kluwer Academic, 2001: 131-40.

NB. The article entitled "Dravet syndrome as epileptic encephalopathy : evidence from long-term course and neuropathology" by Catarino *et al.*, was published in *Brain*, 2011 (Epub, ahead of print), when this book was already in press. We are sorry for being unable to quote the important findings reported in this article at this advanced stage of the printing process.

• Castro MJ, Stam AH, Lemos C, *et al.* First mutation in the voltage-gated Nav1.1 subunit gene SCN1A with co-occurring familial hemiplegic migraine and epilepsy. *Cephalalgia* 2009; 29: 308-13.

• Castro-Gago M, Martinon Sanchez JM, Rodriguez-Nunez A, Herranz Fernandez JL, Eiris-Punal J. Severe myoclonic epilepsy and mitochondrial cytopathy. *Childs Nerv Syst* 1997; 13: 570-1.

• Catterall WA, Dib-Hajj S, Meisler MH, Pietrobon D. Inherited neuronal ion channelopathies: New windows on complex neurological diseases. *J Neurosci* 2008; 28: 11768-77.

• Cestèle S, Scalmani P, Rusconi R, Terragni B, Franceschetti S, Mantegazza M. Self-limited hyperexcitability: Functional effect of a familial hemiplegic migraine mutation of the Nav1.1 (SCN1A) Na+ channel. *J Neurosci* 2008; 28: 7273-83.

• Ceulemans B, Boel M, Claes L, *et al.* Severe myoclonic epilepsy in infancy: towards an optimal treatment. *J Child Neurol* 2004; 19: 516-21.

• Chabardes S, Kahane P, Minotti L, Koudsie A, Hirsch E, Benabid AL. Deep brain stimulation in epilepsy with particular reference to the subthalamic nucleus. *Epileptic Disord* 2002; 4 (Suppl. 3): 83-93.

• Chieffo D, Ricci D, Baranello G, *et al.* Early development in Dravet syndrome; visual function impairment precedes cognitive decline. *Epilepsy Res* 2011a; 93: 73-9.

• Chieffo D, Battaglia D, Lettori D, *et al.* Neuropsychological development in children with Dravet syndrome. *Epilepsy Res* 2011b; 95: 86-93.

• Chipaux M, Villeneuve N, Sabouraud P, *et al.* Unusual consequences of status epilepticus in Dravet syndrome. *Seizure* 2010; 19: 190-4.

• Chiron, C, Marchand, MC, Tran, A, *et al.* Stiripentol in severe myoclonic epilepsy in infancy: A randomized placebo-controlled syndrome-dedicated trial. STICLO study group. *Lancet* 2000; 11: 356: 1638-42.

• Chiron C, Dulac O. The pharmacologic treatment of Dravet Syndrome. *Epilepsia* 2011; 52 (Suppl. 2): 72-5.

• Claes L, Del-Favero J, Ceulemans B, Lagae L, Van Broeckhoven C, De Jonghe P. *De novo* mutations in the sodium-channel gene *SCN1A* cause severe myoclonic epilepsy of infancy. *Am J Hum Genet* 2001; 68: 1327-32.

• Commission on Classification and Terminology of the International League Against Epilepsy. Proposal for revised classification of epilepsies and epileptic syndromes. *Epilepsia* 1989; 30: 289-99.

• Coppola, G, Capovilla, G, Montagnini, A, *et al.* Topiramate as add-on drug in severe myoclonic epilepsy in infancy: An Italian multicenter open trial. *Epilepsy Res* 2002; 49: 45-8.

• Dalla Bernardina B, Capovilla G, Gattoni MB, Colamaria V, Bondavalli S, Bureau M. Épilepsie myoclonique grave de la première année. *Rev EEG Neurophysiol* 1982; 12: 21-5.

• Dalla Bernardina B, Colamaria V, Capovilla G, Bondavalli S. Nosological classification of epilepsies in the first three years of life. In: Nistico G, Di Perri R, Meinardi H (eds). *Epilepsy: an Update on Research and Therapy.* New-York: Alan Liss, 1983: 165-83.

• Dalla Bernardina B, Capovilla G, Chiamenti C, Trevisan E, Colamaria V, Fontana E. Cryptogenic myoclonic epilepsies of infancy and early childhood: Nosological and prognostic approach. In: Wolf P, Dam M, Janz D, Dreifuss FE (eds). *Advances in Epileptology.* New-York: Raven Press, 1987: 175-80.

• Davidsson J, Collin A, Olsson ME, Lundgren J, Soller M. Deletion of the SCN gene cluster on 2q24.4 is associated with severe epilepsy: An array-based genotype-phenotype correlation and a comprehensive review of previously published cases. *Epilepsy Res* 2008; 81: 69-79.

• Delgado-Escueta AV, Bourgeois BF. Debate: Does genetic information in humans help us to treat patients? PRO-genetic information in humans helps us treat patients. CON-genetic information does not help at all. *Epilepsia* 2008; 49 (Suppl. 9): 13-24.

• Delogu AB, Spinelli A, Battaglia D, *et al.* Electrical and autonomic cardiac function in patients affected by Dravet syndrome. *Epilepsia* 2011; 52 (Suppl. 2): 55-8.

• Depienne C, Arzimanoglou A, Trouillard O, *et al.* Parental mosaïcism can cause recurrent transmission of *SCN1A* mutations associated with severe myoclonic epilepsy of infancy. *Hum Mutat* 2006; 27: 389.

• Depienne C, Trouillard O, Saint-Martin C, *et al.* Spectrum of SCN1A gene mutations associated with Dravet syndrome: Analysis of 33 patients. *J Med Genet* 2009a; 46: 183-91.

• Depienne C, Bouteiller D, Keren B, *et al.* Sporadic infantile epileptic encephalopathy caused by mutations in PCDH19 resembles Dravet syndrome but mainly affects females. *PLoS Genet* 2009b; 5: e1000381.

• Depienne C, Trouillard O, Gourfinkel-An I, *et al.* Mechanisms for variable expressivity of inherited SCN1A mutations causing Dravet syndrome. *J Med Genet* 2010; 47: 404-10.

• Dibbens LM, Tarpey PS, Hynes K, *et al.* X-linked protocadherin 19 mutations cause female-limited epilepsy and cognitive impairment. *Nat Genet* 2008; 40: 776-81.

• Dichgans M, Freilinger T, Eckstein G, *et al.* Mutation in the neuronal voltage-gated sodium channel SCN1A in familial hemiplegic migraine. *Lancet* 2005; 366: 371-7.

• Donner EJ, Smith CR, Snead OC[3rd]. Sudden unexplained death in children with epilepsy. *Neurology* 2001; 57: 430-4.

• Dooley J, Camfield P, Gordon K. Severe polymorphic epilepsy of infancy. *J. Child Neurol* 1995; 10: 339-40.

• Doose H, Lunau H, Castiglione E, Waltz S. Severe idiopathic generalized epilepsy of infancy with generalized tonic-clonic seizures. *Neuropediatrics* 1998; 29: 229-38.

• Dravet C. Les épilepsies graves de l'enfant. *Vie Med* 1978; 8: 543-8.

• Dravet C, Dalla Bernardina B, Mesdjian E, Galland MC, Roger J. Dyskinésies paroxystiques au cours des traitements par la diphénylhydantoïne. *Rev Neurol* 1980; 136: 1-14.

• Dravet C, Roger J, Bureau M, Dalla Bernardina B. Myoclonic epilepsies in childhood. In: Akimoto H, *et al.* (eds). *Advances in Epileptology, the XIIIth EIS.* New-York: Raven Press, 1982: 135-40.

• Dravet C, Dalla Bernardina B, Mesdjian E, Galland MC, Roger J. Phenytoin-induced paroxysmal dyskinesias. In: Oxley J, *et al.* (eds). *Antiepileptic Therapy: Chronic Toxicity of Antiepileptic Drugs.* New-York: Raven Press, 1983: 229-35.

• Dravet C, Bureau M, Roger J. Severe myoclonic epilepsy in infancy. In: Roger J, Dravet C, Bureau M, Dreifuss FE, Wolf P (eds). *Epileptic Syndromes in Infancy, Childhood and Adolescence.* London: John Libbey, 1985: 58-67.

• Dravet C, Bureau M, Guerrini R, Giraud N, Roger J. Severe myoclonic epilepsy in infants. In: Roger J, Bureau M, Dravet C, Dreifuss FE, Perret A, Wolf P (eds). *Epileptic Syndromes in Infancy, Childhood and Adolescence* (2nd edition). London: John Libbey, 1992a: 75-88.

• Dravet C, Bureau M, Genton P. Benign myoclonic epilepsy of infancy: electroclinical symptomatology and differential diagnosis from the other types of generalized epilepsy in infancy. In: Degen R, Dreifuss FE (eds). *Epilepsy Research (Suppl. 6), The Benign Localized and Generalized Epilepsies in Early Childhood.* Amsterdam: Elsevier Science, 1992b: 131-5.

• Dravet C, Bureau M, Oguni H, Fukuyama Y, Cokar O. Severe myoclonic epilepsy in infancy (Dravet syndrome). In: Roger J, Bureau M, Dravet C, Genton P, Tassinari CA, Wolf P (eds). *Epileptic syndromes in infancy, childhood and adolescence* (3rd edition), London: John Libbey, 2002: 81-103.

• Dravet C, Bureau M, Oguni H, Fukuyama Y, Cokar O. Severe myoclonic epilepsy in infancy (Dravet Syndrome). In: Roger J, Bureau M, Dravet C, Genton P, Tassinari CA, Wolf P (eds). *Epileptic Syndromes in Infancy, Childhood and Adolescence* (4th edition). Paris: John Libbey Eurotext, 2005a: 89-113.

• Dravet C, Bureau M, Oguni H, Fukuyama Y, Cokar O. Severe myoclonic epilepsy in infancy: Dravet syndrome. In: Delgado-Escueta AV, Guerrini R, Medina MT, Genton P, Bureau M, Dravet C (eds). *Advances in Neurology. Vol. 95.* Philadelphia: Lippincott Williams & Wilkins, 2005b: 71-102.

• Dravet C, Bureau M. Benign myoclonic epilepsy in infancy. In: Roger J, Bureau M, Dravet C, Genton P, Tassinari CA, Wolf P (eds). *Epileptic Syndromes in Infancy, Childhood and Adolescence* (4th edition). Paris: John Libbey Eurotext, 2005: 77-88.

• Dravet C, Daquin G, Battaglia D. Severe myoclonic epilepsy of infancy (Dravet syndrome). In: Nikanorova M, Genton P, Sabers A (eds). *Long-term evolution of epileptic encephalopathies.* Paris: John Libbey Eurotext, 2009: 29-38.

• Dressler A, Stöcklin B, Reithofer E, *et al.* Long-term outcome and tolerability of the ketogenic diet in drug-resistant childhood epilepsy- The Austrian experience. *Seizure* 2010; 19: 404-8.

• Dulac O, Arthuis M. L'épilepsie myoclonique sévère de l'enfant. In : *Journées parisiennes de pédiatrie.* Paris: Flammarion, 1982: 259-68.

• Dura-Trave T, Yoldi-Petri ME, Gallinas-Victoriano F. Epilepsy in children in Navarre, Spain: epileptic seizure types and epileptic syndromes. *J Child Neurol* 2007; 22: 823-8.

• Engel J, Jr. A proposed diagnostic scheme for people with epileptic seizures and with epilepsy. Report of the

ILAE Task Force on Classification and Terminology. *Epilepsia* 2001; 42: 796-803.

• Escayg A, MacDonald BT, Meisler MH, *et al.* Mutations of SCN1A, encoding a neuronal sodium channel, in two families with GEFS+2. *Nat Genet* 2000; 24: 343-5.

• Fisher JL. The anticonvulsant stiripentol acts directly on the $GABA_A$ receptor as a positive allosteric modulator. *Neuropharmacology* 2009; 56: 190-7.

• Fisher JL. Interactions between modulators of the $GABA_A$ receptor: Stiripentol and benzodiazepines. *Eur J Pharmaco* 2011a; 2: 160-5.

• Fisher JL. The effects of stiripentol on $GABA_A$ receptors. *Epilepsia* 2011b; 52 (Suppl. 2): 76-8.

• Fontana E, Dalla Bernardina B, Sgrò V, *et al.* Epilessia mioclonica severa (EMS) e/o sindrome di Dravet: Studio elettroclinico longitudinale di 53 soggetti. *Boll Lega It Epil* 2004; 125/126: 337-40.

• Fujiwara T, Nakamura H, Watanabe M, *et al.* Clinicoelectrographic concordance between monozygotic twins with severe myoclonic epilepsy in infancy. *Epilepsia* 1990; 31: 281-6.

• Fujiwara T, Watanabe M, Takahashi Y, *et al.* Long-term course of childhood epilepsy with intractable Grand Mal seizures. *Jpn J Psychiatr Neurol* 1992; 46: 29.

• Fujiwara T, Sugawara T, Mazaki-Miyazaki E, *et al.* Mutations of sodium channel alpha subunit type 1 *(SCN1A)* in intractable childhood epilepsies with frequent generalized tonic-clonic seizures. *Brain* 2003; 126: 531-46.

• Fukuma G, Oguni H, Shirasaka Y, *et al.* Mutations of neuronal voltage-gated Na+ channel alpha 1 subunit gene SCN1A in core severe myoclonic epilepsy in infancy (SMEI) and in borderline SMEI (SMEB). *Epilepsia* 2004; 45: 140-8.

• Gargus JJ, Tournay A. Novel mutation confirms seizure locus SCN1A is also familial hemiplegic migraine locus FHM3. *Pediatr Neurol* 2007; 37: 407-10.

• Gastaut H, Broughton R, Tassinari CA. Unilateral epileptic seizures. In: Vinken PJ, Bruyn GW (eds). *Handbook of Clinical Neurology: The Epilepsies, Vol. XV*. Amsterdam/New-York: Elsevier, 1974: 235-45.

• Gennaro E, Veggiotti P, Malacarne M, *et al.* Familial severe myoclonic epilepsy of infancy: Truncation of Nav1.1 and genetic heterogeneity. *Epileptic Disord* 2003; 5: 21-5.

• Gennaro E, Santorelli FM, Bertini E, *et al.* Somatic and germline mosaïcisms in Severe myoclonic epilepsy of infancy. *Biochem Biophysl Res Commun* 2006; 341: 489-93.

• Genton P, Velizarova R, Dravet C. Dravet syndrome: The long-term outcome. *Epilepsia* 2011; 52 (Suppl. 2): 44-9.

• Giovanardi-Rossi PR, Santucci M, Gobbi G, Parmeggiani A, Pini A, Ambrosetto G. Long-term follow-up of severe myoclonic epilepsy in infancy. In: Fukuyama Y, Kamoshita S, Ohtsuka C, Susuki Y (eds). *Modern perspectives of child neurology.* Tokyo: Asahi Daily News, 1991: 205-13.

• Giraud C, Treluyer JM, Rey E, *et al.* In vitro and in vivo inhibitory effect of stiripentol on clobazam metabolism. *Drug Metab Dispos* 2006; 34: 608-11.

• Gobbi G, Giovannini S, Boni A, Visconti P, Beghi M, Cornaggia CM. Catatonic psychosis related to forced normalization in a girl with Dravet's syndrome. *Epileptic Disord* 2008; 10: 125-9.

• Goorhuis JF, Verkade HJ, Brouwer OF. Acute hepatic injury in a child with Dravet syndrome: No protective effect of stiripentol. *Seizure* 2008; 17: 477-8.

• Granata T. Comprehensive care of children with Dravet syndrome. *Epilepsia* 2011; 52 (Suppl. 2): 90-4.

• Grosso S, Galimberti D, Farnetani MA, *et al.* Efficacy and safety of topiramate in infants according to epilepsy syndromes. *Seizure* 2005; 14: 183-9.

• Grusser Cornehls U, Baurle J. Mutant mice as a model for cerebellar ataxia. *Progr Neurobiol* 2001; 63: 489-540.

• Guerrini R, Dravet C, Genton P, *et al.* Lamotrigine and seizure aggravation in severe myoclonic epilepsy. *Epilepsia* 1998; 39: 508-12.

• Guerrini R, Pons G (eds). *Comparative Study of the Efficacy of Stiripentol used in Combination in Severe Myoclonic Epilepsy in Infancy (SMEI). A Double-Blind, Multicenter, Placebo-Controlled Phase III Study.* Calambrone (Pisa), Italy: Università di Pisa-IRCCS Stella Maris, 2000.

• Guerrini, R, Tonnelier, S, D'Athis, P, *et al.* Stiripentol in severe myoclonic epilepsy in infancy (SMEI): A placebo-controlled trial. *Epilepsia* 2002; 43 (Suppl. 9): S155.

• Guerrini R, Parmeggiani L, Bonanni P, Kaminska A, Dulac O. Myoclonic astatic epilepsy. In: Roger J, Bureau M, Dravet C, Genton P, Tassinari CA, Wolf P (eds). *Epi-*

leptic Syndromes in Infancy, Childhood and Adolescence (4th edition), Paris: John Libbey Eurotext, 2005: 115-24.

• Guerrini R, Cellini E, Mei D, *et al.* Variable epilepsy phenotypes associated with a familial intragenic deletion of the SCN1A gene. *Epilepsia* 2010; 51: 2474-7.

• Guerrini R, Falchi M. Dravet syndrome and SCN1A gene mutation related-epilepsies: Cognitive impairment and its determinants. *Dev Med Child Neurol* 2011; 53 (Suppl. 2): 11-5.

• Guerrini R, Oguni H. Borderline Dravet syndrome: A useful diagnostic category? *Epilepsia* 2011a; 52 (Suppl. 2): 10-2.

• Guerrini R, Striano P, Catarino C, Sisodiya SM. Neuroimaging and neuropathology of Dravet syndrome. *Epilepsia* 2011b; 52 (Suppl. 2): 30-4.

• Guzzetta F, Cioni G, Mercuri E, *et al.* Neurodevelopmental evolution of West syndrome: A 2-year prospective study. *Eur J Paediatr Neurol* 2008; 12: 387-97

• Harkin LA, Bowser DN, Dibbens LM, *et al.* Truncation of the GABA(A)-receptor gamma2 subunit in a family with generalized epilepsy with febrile seizures plus. *Am J Hum Genet* 2002; 70: 530-53.

• Harkin LA, McMahon JM, Iona X, *et al.* The spectrum of SCN1A-related infantile epileptic encephalopathies. *Brain* 2007; 130: 843-52.

• Hartman AL, Vining EPG. Clinical aspects of the ketogenic diet. *Epilepsia* 2007; 48: 31-42.

• Hattori J, Ouchida M, Ono J, *et al.* A screening test for the prediction of Dravet syndrome before one year of age. *Epilepsia* 2008; 49: 626-33.

• Hayashi M, Sugai K, Kurihara E, Tamagawa K. An Autopsy Case of Severe Myoclonic Epilepsy of Infancy, Who Died of Acute Encephalopathy Associated with Influenza Infection. *Epilepsia* 2004; 45 (Suppl. 8): 65.

• Hino-Fukuyo N, Haginoya K, Togashi N, *et al.* Ictal vomiting as an initial symptom of Severe myoclonic epilepsy in infancy: A case report. *J Child Neurol* 2009; 24: 228.

• Horn CS, Ater SB, Hurst DL. Carbamazepine-exacerbated epilepsy in children and adolescents. *Pediatr Neurol* 1986; 2: 340-5.

• Hurst DL. Epidemiology of severe myoclonic epilepsy of infancy. *Epilepsia* 1990; 31: 397-400.

• Hurst DL. Severe myoclonic epilepsy in infancy. *Pediatr Neurol* 1987; 3: 269-72.

• Ianetti P, Parisi P, Spalice A, Ruggieri M, Zara F. Addition of verapamil in the treatment of severe myoclonic epilepsy in infancy. *Epilepsy Res* 2009; 85: 89-95.

• Inoue Y, Ohtsuka Y, Oguni H, *et al.* Stiripentol open study in Japanese patients with Dravet Syndrome. *Epilepsia* 2009: 50: 2362-8.

• Jansen FE, Sadleir LG, Harkin LA, *et al.* Severe myoclonic epilepsy of infancy (Dravet syndrome): Recognition and diagnosis in adults. *Neurology* 2006; 67: 224-6.

• Kalume F, Yu FH, Westenbroek RE, Scheuer T, Catterall WA. Reduced sodium current in Purkinje neurons from Nav1.1 mutant mice: implications for ataxia in severe myoclonic epilepsy in infancy. *J Neurosci* 2007; 27: 11065-74.

• Kanazawa O. Medically intractable generalized tonic-clonic or clonic seizures in infancy. *J Epil* 1992; 5: 143-8.

• Kanazawa O, Shirane S. Can early zonizamide medication improve the prognosis in the core and peripheral types of severe myoclonic epilepsy in infants? *Brain Dev* 1999; 21: 503.

• Kassai B, Chiron C, Augier S, *et al.* Severe myoclonic epilepsy in infancy: A systematic review and a meta-analysis of individual patient data. *Epilepsia* 2008; 49: 343-8.

• Kearney JA, Wiste AK, Stephani U, *et al.* Recurrent *de novo* mutations of *SCN1A* in Severe myoclonic epilepsy of infancy. *Pediatr Neurol* 2006; 34, 2: 116-20.

• Kimura K, Sugawara T, Mazaki-Miyazaki E, *et al.* A missense mutation in *SCN1A* in brothers with severe myoclonic epilepsy in infancy (SMEI) inherited from a father with febrile seizures. *Brain Dev* 2005; 27: 424-30.

• Korff C, Laux L, Kelley K, Goldstein J, Koh S, Nordli D Jr. Dravet syndrome (Severe myoclonic epilepsy in infancy): A retrospective study of 16 patients. *J Child Neurol* 2007; 22: 185-94.

• Kossoff EH, Zupec-Kania BA, Amark PE, *et al.* Optimal clinical management of children receiving the ketogenic diet: Recommendations of the International Ketogenic Diet Study Group. *Epilepsia* 2009; 50: 304-17.

• Krishna-K K, Hertel N, Redies C. Cadherin expression in the somatosensory cortex: Evidence for a combinatorial molecular code at the single-cell level. *Neuroscience* 2011; 175: 37-48.

• Kroll-Seger J, Portilla P, Dulac O, *et al.* Topiramate in the treatment of highly refractory patients with Dravet syndrome. *Neuropediatrics* 2006; 37: 325-9.

• Lambarri San Martin I, Garaizar Axpe C, Zuazo Zamalloa E, *et al.* Epilepsia polimorfa de la infancia: revision de 12 casos. *Anales Españoles de Pediatria* 1997; 46: 571-5.

• Le Gal F, Korff CM, Monso-Hinard C, *et al.* A case of SUDEP in a patient with Dravet syndrome with SCN1A mutation. *Epilepsia* 2010; 51: 1915-8.

• Liu X, Muller RU, Huang LT, *et al.* Seizure-induced changes in place cell physiology: Relationship to spatial memory. *J Neurosci* 2003; 23: 11505-15.

• Madia F, Striano P, Gennaro E, *et al.* Cryptic chromosome deletions involving SCN1A in severe myoclonic epilepsy of infancy. *Neurology* 2006; 67: 1230-5.

• Mancardi M, Striano P, Gennaro E, *et al.* Familial occurrence of febrile seizures and epilepsy in severe myoclonic epilepsy of infancy (SMEI) patients with *SCN1A* mutations. *Epilepsia* 2006; 47: 1629-35.

• Mangano S, Fontana A, Cusumano L. Benign myoclonic epilepsy in infancy: Neuropsychological and behavioral outcome. *Brain Dev* 2005; 27: 218-23.

• Marini C, Mei D, Cross JH, Guerrini R. Mosaic SCN1A mutation in familial severe myoclonic epilepsy of infancy. *Epilepsia* 2006; 47: 1737-40.

• Marini C, Mei D, Temudo T, *et al.* Idiopathic epilepsies with seizures precipitated by fever and *SCN1A* abnormalities. *Epilepsia* 2007; 48: 1678-96.

• Marini C, Scheffer IE, Nabbout R, *et al.* SCN1A duplications and deletions detected in Dravet syndrome: implications for molecular diagnosis. *Epilepsia* 2009; 50: 1670-8.

• Marini C, Mei D, Parmeggiani L, *et al.* Protocadherin 19 mutations in girls with infantile-onset epilepsy. *Neurology* 2010; 75: 646-53.

• Martin MS, Dutt K, Papale LA, *et al.* Altered function of the SCN1A voltage-gated sodium channel leads to gamma-aminobutyric acid-ergic (GABAergic) interneuron abnormalities. *J Biol Chem* 2010; 285: 9823-34.

• McGregor A, Wheeless J. Pediatric experience with sudden unexplained death in epilepsy at a tertiary center. *J Child Neurol* 2006; 21: 782-7.

• McIntosh AM, McMahon J, Dibbens LM, Iona X, Mulley JC, Scheffer IE, Berkovic SF. Effects of vaccination on onset and outcome of Dravet syndrome: A retrospective study. *Lancet Neurol* 2010; 9: 559-61.

• McMullan J, Sasson C, Pancioli A, Silbergleit R. Midazolam versus diazepam for the treatment of status epilepticus in children and young adults: a meta-analysis. *Acad Emerg Med* 2010; 17: 575-82.

• Meisler MH, Kearney JA. Sodium channel mutations in epilepsy and other neurological disorders. *J Clin Invest* 2005; 115: 2010-7.

• Mercuri E, Haataja L, Guzzetta A, *et al.* Visual function in term infants with hypoxic-ischemic insults; correlation with neurodevelopment at 2 years of age. *Arch Dis Child Fetal Neonatal Ed* 1999; 80: F99-104.

• Miyama S, Goto T, Inoue Y, Yamakawa K. Monozygotic twins with severe myoclonic epilepsy in infancy discordant for clinical features. *Pediatr Neurol* 2008; 39: 120-2.

• Miyamoto A, Itoh M, Hayashi K, Hara M, Fukuyama Y. Diurnal secretion profile of melatonin in epileptic children with or without photosensitivity and an observation of aletred circadian rhythm in a case of completely under dark living condition. *No To Hattatsu* (in Japanese) 1993; 25: 405-11.

• Morimoto M, Mazaki E, Nishimura A, *et al. SCN1*A mutation mosaïcism in a family with severe myoclonic epilepsy in infancy. *Epilepsia* 2006; 47: 1732-6.

• Mulley JC, Scheffer IE, Petrou S, Dibbens LM, Berkovic SF, Harkin LA. SCN1A mutations and epilepsy. *Hum Mutat* 2005; 25: 535-42.

• Mulley JC, Nelson P, Guerrero S, *et al.* A new molecular mechanism for severe myoclonic epilepsy of infancy: Exonic deletions in SCN1A. *Neurology* 2006; 67: 1094-5.

• Musumeci SA, Elia M, Ferri R, Scuderi C, Schepis C, Bergonzi P. Severe myoclonic epilepsy in two monozygous subjects affected by Rud syndrome. *Boll Lega It Epil* 1992; 79/80: 81-2.

• Nabbout R, Gennaro E, Dalla Bernardina B, *et al.* Spectrum of *SCN1A* mutations in severe myoclonic epilepsy of infancy. *Neurology* 2003; 60: 1961-7.

• Nabbout R, Desguerre I, Sabbagh S, *et al.* An unexpected EEG course in Dravet syndrome. *Epilepsy Res* 2008; 81: 90-5.

• Nabbout R, Copioli C, Chipaux M, *et al.* Ketogenic diet also benefits Dravet syndrome patients receiving stiripentol: A prospective pilot study. *Epilepsia* 2011; 52: 54-7.

• Naegele JR, Vemuri MC, Studer L. Embryonic stem cell therapy for intractable epilepsy. *Epilepsia* 2010; 51 (Suppl. 9): 93.

• Nakayama T, Ogiwara I, Ito K, *et al.* Deletions of SCN1A 5' genomic region with promoter activity in Dravet syndrome. *Hum Mutat* 2010; 31: 820-9.

• Nicolai J, Gunning B, Leroy PL, Ceulemans B, Vies JSH. Acute hepatic injury in four children with Dravet syndrome: Valproic acid, topiramate or acetaminophen? *Seizure* 2008; 17: 92-7.

• Nieto M, Roldan S, Sanchez B, *et al.* Estudio immunológico en pacientes con epilepsia mioclónica severa en la infancia. *Rev Neurol* (Spanish) 2000; 30: 1-15.

• Nieto-Barrera M, Candau R, Rufo, M, Ruiz del Portal L. Epilepsia mioclonica grave de la infancia. Tratamiento con gammaglobulina humana. *Rev Neurol* (Spanish) 1995; 24: 1250-70.

• Nieto-Barrera M, Lillo MM, Rodriguez-Collado C, Candau R, Correa A. Epilepsia mioclonica severa de la infancia. Estudio epidemiologico analitico. *Rev Neurol* (Spanish) 2000a; 30: 620-4.

• Nieto-Barrera M, Candau R, Nieto-Jimenez M, Correa A, del Portal LR. Topiramate in the treatment of severe myoclonic epilepsy in infancy. *Seizure* 2000b; 8: 590-4.

• Nishri D, Blumkin L, Lev D, *et al.* Hepatic coma culminating in severe brain damage in a child with a *SCN1A* mutation. *Eur J Paed Neurol* 2010; 14: 456-9.

• Nolan KJ, Camfield CS, Camfield PR. Coping with Dravet syndrome: Parental experiences with a catastrophic epilepsy. *Dev Med Child Neurol* 2006; 48:761-5.

• Nolan K, Camfield CS, Camfield PR. Coping with a child with Dravet syndrome: Insights from families. *J Child Neurol* 2008; 23: 690-4.

• Ogihara M, Hoshika A, Matsuno T, *et al.* EEG and polygraphical study of vibratory generalized tonic-clonic seizures (vibratory GTCS). *J Jpn Epil Soc* (Japanese) 1994; 12: 264-71.

• Ogino T, Ohtsuka Y, Mimaki N, *et al.* Severe myoclonic epilepsy in infancy. *Folia Psychiatrica et Neurologica Japonica* 1985; 39: 357-8.

• Ogino T. Severe myoclonic epilepsy in infancy – a clinical and electroencephalographic study. *J Jpn Epil Soc* 1986; 4: 114-26.

• Ogino T, Ohtsuka y, Tamatogi Y, *et al.* The epileptic syndrome sharing common characteristics during early childhood with severe myoclonic epilepsy in infancy. *Jpn J Psychiatry Neurol* 1989; 43: 479-81.

• Ogiwara I, Miyamoto H, Morita N, *et al.* Na(v)1.1 localizes to axons of parvalbumin-positive inhibitory interneurons: A circuit basis for epileptic seizures in mice carrying an Scn1a gene mutation. *J Neurosci* 2007; 27: 5903-14.

• Oguni, H, Kitami, H, Oguni, M, *et al.* Treatment of severe myoclonic epilepsy in infants and its borderline variant with bromide. *Epilepsia* 1994; 35: 1140-5.

• Oguni H, Hayashi K, Awaya Y, Fukuyama Y, Osawa M. Severe myoclonic epilepsy in infants – a review based on the Tokyo Women's medical university series of 84 cases. *Brain Dev* 2001; 23: 736-48.

• Oguni H, Hayashi K, Osawa M, *et al.* Severe myoclonic epilepsy in infants. Typical and borderline groups in relation to *SCN1A* mutations. In: Delgado-Escueta V, Guerrini R, Medina MT, Genton P, Bureau M, Dravet C (eds). *Advances in Neurology, vol 95, Myoclonic Epilepsies.* Philadelphia: Lippincott Williams & Wilkins, 2005: 103-11.

• Ohki T, Watanabe K, Negoro K, *et al.* Severe myoclonic epilepsy in infancy: Evolution of seizures. *Seizure* 1997; 6: 219-24.

• Ohmori I, Ohtsuka Y, Murakami N, Asano T, Hattori J, Oka E. Analysis of ictal EEG in Severe Myoclonic Epilepsy in infancy. *Epilepsia* 2001; 42 (suppl 6): 54 (abstr).

• Ohmori I, Ouchida M, Ohtsuka Y, Oka E, Shimizu K. Significant correlation of the *SCN1A* mutations and severe myoclonic epilepsy in infancy. *Biochem Biophys Res Commun* 2002; 295: 17-23.

• Ohmori I, Ohtsuka Y, Ouchida M, Ogino T, Maniwa S, Shimizu K, Oka E. Is phenotype difference in severe myoclonic epilepsy in infancy related to *SCN1A* mutations? *Brain Dev* 2003; 27: 488-93.

• Ohmori I, Ouchida M, Kobayashi K, *et al.* Rasmussen encephalitis associated with SCN1A mutation. *Epilepsia* 2008; 49: 521-6.

• Ohtsuka Y, Maniwa S, Ogino T, Yamatogi Y, Ohtahara S. Severe myoclonic epilepsy in infancy: A long-term follow-up study. *Jpn J Psychiatr Neurol* 1991; 45: 416-8.

• Ohtsuka Y, Ohmori I, Ogino T, Ouchuida M, Shimizu K, Oka E. Paroxysmal movement disorders in seere myoclonic epilepsy in infancy. *Brain Dev* 2003; 25: 401-5.

• Okumura A, Kurahashi H, Hirose S, *et al.* Focal epilepsy resulting from a *de novo SCN1A* mutation. *Neuropediatrics* 2007; 38: 253-6.

• Patino GA, Claes LR, Lopez-Santiago LF, *et al.* A functional null mutation of SCN1B in a patient with Dravet syndrome. *J Neurosci* 2009; 29: 2910764-78.

• Pereira S, Vieira JP, Barroca F, *et al.* Severe epilepsy, retardation, and dysmorphic features with a 2q deletion including SCN1A and SCN2A. *Neurology* 2004; 63: 191-2.

• Prunetti P, Perucca E. New and forthcoming antiepileptic drugs. *Curr Opin Neurol* 2011; 2: 159-64.

• Ragona F, Brazzo D, De Giorgi I, *et al.* Dravet syndrome: Early clinical manifestations and cognitive outcome in 37 Italian patients. *Brain Dev* 2010; 32: 71-7.

• Ragona F, Granata T, Dalla Bernardina B, *et al.* Cognitive development in Dravet syndrome: A retrospective, multi center study of 26 patients. *Epilepsia* 2011; 52: 386-92.

• Ragsdale DS. How do mutant Nav1.1 sodium channels cause epilepsy? *Brain Res Rev* 2008; 58: 149-59.

• Renier WO, Renkawek K. Clinical and neuropathologic findings in a case of severe myoclonic epilepsy of infancy. *Epilepsia* 1990; 31: 287-91.

• Riva D, Vago C, Pantaleoni C, Bulgheroni S, Mantegazza M, Franceschetti S. Progressive neurocognitive decline in two children with Dravet syndrome, de novo SCN1A truncations and different epileptic phenotypes. *Am J Med Genet Part A.* 2009; 149A: 2339-45.

• Sakauchi M, Oguni H, Kato I, *et al.* Mortality in Dravet syndrome: Search for risk factors in Japanese patients. *Epilepsia* 2011; 52 (Suppl. 2): 50-4.

• Sakakibara T, Nakagawa E, Saito Y, *et al.* Hemiconvulsion-hemiplegia syndrome in a patient with severe myoclonic epilepsy in infancy. *Epilepsia* 2009; 50: 2158-62.

• Sarisjulis N, Gamboni B, Plouin P, Kaminska A, Dulac O. Diagnosing idiopathic/cryptogenic epilepsy syndromes in infancy. *Arch Dis Child* 2000; 82: 226-30.

• Saito Y, Oguni H, Awaya Y, Hayashi K, Osawa M. Phenytoin-induced choreoathetosis in patients with severe myoclonic epilepsy in infancy. *Neuropediatrics* 2001; 32: 231-5.

• Sato T, Ota M, Matsuo M, Tasaki H, Miyazaki S. Recurrent reversible rhabdomyolisis associated with hyperthermia and status epilepticus. *Acta Paediatr* 1995 ; 84: 1083-5.

• Scheffer IE, Turner SJ, Dibbens LM, *et al.* Epilepsy and mental retardation limited to females: An under-recognized disorder. *Brain* 2008; 131: 918-27.

• Siegler Z, Barsi P, Neuwirth M, *et al.* Hippocampal sclerosis in severe myoclonic epilepsy in infancy: A retrospective MRI study. *Epilepsia* 2005; 46: 704-8.

• Singh R, Andermann E, Whitehouse WP, *et al.* Severe myoclonic epilepsy of infancy: Extended spectrum of GEFS+? *Epilepsia* 2001; 42: 837-44.

• Singh NA, Pappas C, Dahle EJ, *et al.* A role of SCN9A in human epilepsies, as a cause of febrile seizures and as a potential modifier of Dravet syndrome. *PLoS Genet* 2009; 5: e1000649.

• Skluzacek JV, Watts KP, Parsy O, *et al.* Dravet syndrome and parent associations: The IDEA League experience with comorbid conditions, mortality, management, adaptation, and grief. *Epilepsia* 2011; 52 (Suppl. 2): 95-101.

• Specchio N, Kasteleijn-Nost-Trenité DGA, Piccioli M, *et al.* Diagnosing photosensitive epilepsy: Fancy new versus old fashioned techniques in patients with different epileptic syndromes. *Brain Dev* 2011; 33: 294-300.

• Striano P, Mancardi MM, Biancheri R, *et al.* Brain MRI findings in severe myoclonic epilepsy in infancy and genotype-phenotype correlations. *Epilepsia* 2007a; 48: 1092-6.

• Striano P, Coppola G, Pezella M, *et al.*. An open-label trial of levetiracetam in severe myoclonic epilepsy of infancy. *Neurology* 2007b; 69: 922-5.

• Sugama M, Oguni H, Fukuyama Y. Clinical and electroencephalographic study of severe myoclonic epilepsy in infancy (Dravet). *Jpn J Psychiat Neurol* 1987; 41: 463-5.

• Suls A, Claeys KG, Goossens D, *et al.* Microdeletions involving the SCN1A gene may be common in SCN1A-mutation-negative SMEI patients. *Hum Mutat* 2006; 27: 914-20.

• Suls A, Velizarova R, Yordanova I, *et al.* Four generations of epilepsy caused by an inherited microdeletion of the SCN1A gene. *Neurology* 2010; 75: 72-6.

• Takahashi T, Tsukahara Y. Usefulness of blue sunglasses in photosensitive epilepsy. *Epilepsia* 1992; 33: 517-21.

• Takahashi Y, Shigematsu H, Fujiwara T, Yagi K, Seino M. Self-induced photogenic seizures in a child with severe myoclonic epilepsy in infancy: Optical investigations and treatments. *Epilepsia* 1995; 36: 728-32.

• Takahashi Y, Fujiwara T, Yagi K, Seino M. Photosensitive epilepsies and pathophysiologic mechanisms of the photoparoxysmal response. *Neurology* 1999; 53: 926-32.

• Takayanagi M, Haginoya K, Umehara N, *et al.* Acute encephalopathy with a truncation mutation in the SCN1A gene: A case report. *Epilepsia* 2010; 51: 1886-8.

• Tanabe T, Awaya Y, Matsuishi T, *et al.* Survey of vaccination and viral infections for children with severe myoclonic epilepsy in infancy. *No To Hattatsu* 2004; 36: 318-23.

• Tanabe T, Awaya Y, Matsuishi T, *et al.* Management of and prophylaxis against status epilepticus in children with severe myoclonic epilepsy in infancy (SMEI; Dravet syndrome): A nation-wide questionnaire survey in Japan. *Brain Dev* 2008; 30: 629-35.

• Than TN, Chiron C, Dellatolas G, *et al.* Long-term efficacy and tolerance of Stiripentol in severe myoclonic epilepsy of infancy (Dravet's syndrome). *Arch Pediatr* 2002; 9: 1120-7.

• Tro-Baumann B, von Spiczak S, Lotte J, *et al.* A retrospective study of the relation between vaccination and occurrence of seizures in Dravet syndrome. *Epilepsia* 2011; 52: 175-8.

• Vadlamudi L, Dibbens LM, Lawrence KM, *et al.* Timing of de novo mutagenesis--a twin study of sodium-channel mutations. *N Engl J Med* 2010; 363: 1335-40.

• Vahedi K, Depienne C, Le Fort D, *et al.* Elicited repetitive daily blindness: A new phenotype associated with hemiplegic migraine and SCN1A mutations. *Neurology* 2009; 72: 1178-83.

• Vanmolkot KR, Babini E, de Vries B, *et al.* The novel p.L1649Q mutation in the SCN1A epilepsy gene is associated with familial hemiplegic migraine: Genetic and functional studies. *Hum Mutat* 2007; 28: 522.

• Veggiotti P, Cardinalii S, Montalenti E, Gatti A, Lanzi G. Generalized epilepsy with febrile seizures plus and severe myoclonic epilepsy in infancy: A case report of two Italian families. *Epileptic Disord* 2001; 3: 29-32.

• Veggiotti P, Burlina A, Coppola G, *et al.* The ketogenic diet for Dravet syndrome and other epileptic encephalopathies: An Italian consensus. *Epilepsia* 2011; 52 (Suppl. 2): 83-9.

• Villeneuve N, Portilla P, Ferrari AR, *et al.* Topiramate (TPM) in severe myoclonic epilepsy in infancy (SMEI): Study of 27 patients. *Epilepsia* 2002; 43 (Suppl 8): 155.

• Wakai S, Ikehata M, Nihira H, *et al.* "Obtundation status (Dravet)" caused by complex partial status epilepticus in a patient with severe myoclonic epilepsy in infancy. *Epilepsia* 1996a; 37: 1020-2.

• Wakai S, Ito N, Sueoka H, *et al.* Severe myoclonic epilepsy in infancy and carbamazepine. *Eur J Pediatr* 1996b; 155: 724.

• Wallace SJ. Myoclonus and epilepsy in childhood: A review of treatment with valproate, ethosuximide, lamotrigine and zonizamide. *Epilepsy Res* 1998; 29: 147-54.

• Wallace RH, Hodgson BL, Grinton BE, *et al.* Sodium channel alpha1-subunit mutations in severe myoclonic epilepsy of infancy and infantile spasms. *Neurology* 2003; 61: 765-9.

• Wang PJ, Fan PC, Lee WT, Young C, Huang CC, Shen YZ. Severe myoclonic epilepsy in infancy: evolution of electroencephalographic and clinical features. *Acta Paed Sin* 1996; 37: 428-32.

• Wang JW, Kurahashi H, Ishii A, *et al.* Microchromosomal deletions involving SCN1A and adjacent genes in severe myoclonic epilepsy in infancy. *Epilepsia* 2008; 49: 1528-34.

• Wical B, Leighty D, Wendorf H, Tervo M, Tervo R, Maytum J. Signs of dysautonomia in children with Dravet syndrome (abstract). *Epilepsia* 2009; 50 (Suppl. 3): 164.

• Wolff M, Cassé-Perrot C, Dravet C. Severe myoclonic epilepsy of infants (Dravet syndrome): Natural history and neuropsychological findings. *Epilepsia* 2006; 47 (Suppl. 2): 45-8.

• Yagi T, Takeichi M. Cadherin superfamily genes: Function, genomic organization, and neurologic diversity. *Genes Dev* 2000; 14: 1169-80.

• Yakoub LM, Dulac O, Jambaqué I, Plouin P. Early diagnosis of severe myoclonic epilepsy in infancy. *Brain Dev* 1992; 14: 299-303.

• Yasuda S, Watanabe M, Fujiwara T, Yagi K, Seino M. A peculiar state observed in 4 patients with severe myoclonic epilepsy in infancy. *Jpn J Psycchiatr Neurol* 1989; 43: 533-5.

• Yu FH, Mantegazza M, Westenbroek RE, *et al.* Reduced sodium current in GABAergic interneurons in a mouse model of severe myoclonic epilepsy in infancy. *Nat Neurosci* 2006; 9: 1142-9.

• Zaatreh M, Tennison M, D'Cruz O, Beach RL. Anticonvulsants-induced chorea: A role for pharmacodynamic drug interaction? *Seizure* 2001; 10: 596-9.

• Zamponi N, Passamonti C, Cappanera S, Petrelli C. Clinical course of young patients with Dravet syndrome after vagal nerve stimulation. *Eur J Ped Neurol* 2010; 30: 1-7.

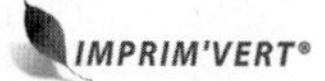

Achevé d'imprimer par Corlet, Imprimeur, S.A.
14110 Condé-sur-Noireau
N° d'Imprimeur : 139464 - Dépôt légal : août 2011
Imprimé en France